Weapons of Mass Destruction
Emergency Care

Robert A. De Lorenzo, MD, FACEP

Major, Medical Corps, Flight Surgeon, US Army
US Army Academy of Health Sciences
Ft. Sam Houston, Texas

Clinical Associate Professor of Military
and Emergency Medicine
Uniformed Services University of the Health Sciences
Bethesda, Maryland

Robert S. Porter, MA, EMT-P, Flight Paramedic

Senior Advanced Life Support Educator, Madison County EMS
Hamilton, NY

Flight Paramedic, AirOne, Onondaga County Sherif Department
Syracuse, NY

D0207170

Brady
Prentice Hall Health
Upper Saddle River, New Jersey 07458

Library of Congress Cataloging-in-Publication Data

De Lorenzo, Robert A.

    Weapons of mass destruction: emergency care /
Robert A. De Lorenzo, Robert S. Porter.

      p.   cm.

    Includes bibliographical references and index.

    ISBN 0-13-013923-8 (alk. paper)

    1. Terrorism--Health aspects--Handbooks, manuals, etc. 2. Weapons
of mass destruction--Health aspects--Handbooks, manuals, etc.
3. Disaster medicine--Handbooks, manuals, etc. 4. First aid in
illness and injury--Handbooks, manuals, etc. I. Porter, Robert S.,
1950- . II. Title.

RC88.9.T47D4 1999

616.02'5--dc21   98-50344

                                             CIP

Publisher: Julie Alexander
Acquisitions Editor: Sherene Miller
Editorial Assistant: Jean Molenaar
Marketing Manager: Tiffany Price
Marketing Coordinator: Cindy Frederick
Director of Production and Manufacturing: Bruce Johnson
Managing Production Editor: Patrick Walsh
Senior Production Manager: Ilene Sanford
Production Editor: Larry Hayden IV
Creative Director: Marianne Frasco
Cover design: Miguel Ortiz
Composition: Lido Graphics
Presswork and Binding: R.R. Donnelley, Harrisonburg, Virginia

©2000 by Prentice-Hall, Inc.
A Pearson Education Company
Upper Saddle River, New Jersey 07458

Printed in the United States of America

10 9 8 7 6 5 4 3 2 1

ISBN 0-13-013923-8

Prentice-Hall International (UK) Limited, *London*
Prentice-Hall of Australia Pty., Limited, *Sydney*
Prentice-Hall Canada Inc., *Toronto*
Prentice-Hall Hispanoamericana, S.A., *Mexico*
Prentice-Hall of India Private Limited, *New Delhi*
Prentice-Hall of Japan, Inc., *Tokyo*
Prentice-Hall (Singapore) Pte. Ltd
Editoria Prentice-Hall do Brasil, Ltda., *Rio de Janeiro*

Contents

Preface

This handbook is designed to help the emergency care provider deal with the medical consequences of terrorist attacks. In particular, this book will address the prehospital emergency care of victims of conventional bombings, incendiary attacks, chemical and biological agents, and nuclear devices. The goal is to provide a rational medical approach to the care of casualties of weapons of mass destruction. This book is directed at prehospital care providers of all levels of training. Sufficient depth and breadth is provided to appeal to physicians, nurses, allied health personnel and administrators and planners as well. Material for this book was synthesized from multiple sources, including military and civilian references. The result is the best of both.

The authors endeavor to provide the best and most up-to-date information available. Readers wishing to suggest new or improved material are invited to contact the authors through the publisher.

R.A.D. & R.S.P.

NOTICES

Drugs and Drug Dosages

Every effort has been made to ensure that the drug dosages presented in this textbook are in accordance with nationally accepted standards. When applicable, the dosages and routes are taken from the American Heart Association's Advanced Cardiac Life Support Guidelines. The American Medical Association's publication *Drug Evaluations*, and the material published in the *Physician's Desk Reference*, are followed with regard to drug dosages not covered by the American Heart Association's guidelines. It is the responsibility of the reader to be familiar with the drugs used in his or her system, as well as the dosages specified by the medical director. The drugs presented in this book should only be administered by direct order, either verbally or through accepted standing orders, of a licensed physician.

Gender Usage

The English language has historically given preference to the male gender. Among many words, the pronouns "he" and "his" are commonly used to describe both genders. Society evolves faster than language and the male pronouns still predominate in our speech. The authors have made great effort to treat the two genders equally, recognizing that a significant percentage of paramedics are female. However, in some instances, male pronouns may be used to describe both male and female paramedics solely for the purpose of brevity. This is not intended to offend any readers of the female gender.

Photographs

Please note that many of the photographs contained in this book are taken of actual emergency situations. As such, it is possible that they may not accurately depict current, appropriate, or advisable practices of emergency medical care. They have been included for the sole purpose of giving general insight into real-life emergency settings.

Body Substance Isolation Precautions and Personal Protective Equipment

Emergency response personnel should practice Body Substance Isolation (BSI), a strategy that considers ALL body substances potentially infectious. To achieve this, all emergency personnel should utilize personal protective equipment (PPE). Appropriate PPE should be available on every emergency vehicle. The minimum recommended PPE includes the following.

- **Gloves.** Disposable gloves should be donned by all emergency response personnel BEFORE initiating any emergency care. When an emergency incident involves more than one patient, you should attempt to change gloves between patients. When gloves have been contaminated, they should be removed as soon as possible. To properly remove contaminated gloves, grasp one glove approximately one inch from the wrist. Without touching the inside of the glove, pull the glove half-way off and stop. With that half gloved hand, pull the glove on the opposite hand completely off. Place the removed glove in the palm of the other glove, with the inside of the removed glove exposed. Pull the second glove completely off with the ungloved hand, only touching the inside of the glove. Always wash hands after gloves are removed, even when the gloves appear intact.

- **Masks and Protective Eyewear.** Masks and protective equipment should be present on all emergency vehicles and used in accordance with the level of exposure encountered. Masks and protective eyewear should be worn together whenever blood spatter is likely to occur, such as arterial bleeding, childbirth, endotracheal intubation, invasive procedures, oral suctioning, and clean-up of equipment that requires heavy scrubbing or brushing. Both you and the patient should wear masks whenever the potential for airborne transmission of disease exists.

- **HEPA Respirators.** Due to the resurgence of tuberculosis (TB), prehospital personnel should protect themselves from TB infection through use of a high-efficiency particulate air (HEPA) respirator, a design approved by the National Institute of Occupational Safety and Health (NIOSH). It should fit snugly and be capable of filtering out the tuberculosis bacillus. The HEPA respirator should be worn when caring for patients with confirmed or suspected TB. This is especially true when performing "high hazard" procedures such as administration of nebulized medications, endotracheal intubation, or suctioning on such a patient.

- **Gowns.** Gowns protect clothing from blood splashes. If large splashes of blood are expected, such as with childbirth, wear impervious gowns.
- **Resuscitation Equipment.** Disposable resuscitation equipment should be the primary means of artificial ventilation in emergency care. Such items should be used once, then disposed of.

Remember, the proper use of personal protective equipment ensures effective infection control and minimizes risk. Use ALL protective equipment recommended for any particular situation to ensure maximum protection. Consider ALL body substances potentially infectious and ALWAYS practice body substance isolation.

Department of Defense

The opinions or assertions in this text are solely the authors' and do not necessarily represent the official views of the Department of Defense.

AUTHOR BIOS

Robert A. De Lorenzo, MD, FACEP

Robert A. De Lorenzo, MD, FACEP is a major in the US Army on active duty. He has over 18 years experience in traditional EMS settings, including basic EMT, paramedic, training officer, and medical director. He is also expert in military medicine and specializes in tactical emergency medicine. He is author of the textbook *Tactical Emergency Care* numerous EMS and military articles in the medical peer-review and EMS literature.

Robert S. Porter, MA, EMT-P

Robert S. Porter, MA, EMT-P is the Senior Advanced Life Support Educator for Madison County, New York and a flight paramedic with AirOne, of the Onondaga County Sheriff's Department. He is coauthor of the successful Brady series of EMS textbooks including *Tactical Emergency Care*, *Paramedic Emergency Care*, and *Intermediate Emergency Care*. He has over 25 years of EMS education and administrative experience and is considered a national leader in EMS education.

DEDICATION

This book is dedicated to the brave young men and women of EMS who tirelessly serve their communities by providing the very best emergency care.

ACKNOWLEDGMENTS

The authors are grateful to many people for making this project successful. First and foremost, I (RAD) thank my wife, Karen De Lorenzo, for her unyielding support and unwavering love. Also, many thanks to the Brady staff and leadership, and in particular Sherene Miller and Susan Katz. We also gratefully acknowledge the technical expertise of the following individuals, many of whom also reviewed material for the parent text *Tactical Emergency Care*.

Special thanks to the following individuals for their expert review of the concept and content of this textbook. Their efforts were instrumental in shaping the final form of this book. Their appearance here does not constitute endorsement by their respective agencies.

KEVIN YESKEY, MD, FACEP
Cmdr, US Public Health Service
Department of Military and Emergency Medicine
Uniformed Services University of the Health Sciences
Bethesda, MD 20814-4799

JEFF T. DYAR
Chair, EMS Programs
National Fire Academy
Emmitsburg, MD 21727

The authors are grateful to the following individuals who shared their time and expertise in helping integrate the wealth of material in this book. They are acknowledged experts in their fields and provided invaluable technical advice. Their appearance here does not constitute endorsement by their respective agencies.

COL. JAMES A. PFAFF, MD, FACEP
Brooke Army Medical Center
Ft. Sam Houston, TX

Sgt. 1st Class ROBERT MALLOY, EMT-P
US Army Medical Department Center and School
Ft. Sam Houston, TX

Cmdr. JERRY MOTHERSHEAD, MD, FACEP
Naval Medical Center
Portsmouth Naval Base, VA

Sgt. 1st Class DAVID A. SCOTT, LPN, EMT

US Army Medical Department Center and School
Ft. Sam Houston, TX

Cmdr. GARRY B. CRIDDLE, RN
US Coast Guard/Public Health Service
Washington, DC

Capt. STEVEN W. SALYER, PhD, PA-C
Brooke Army Medical Center
Ft. Sam Houston, TX

JON R. KROHMER, MD, FACEP
Kent County EMS
Grand Rapids, MI

Col. CRAIG H. LLEWELLYN, MD, MPH, US Army (Ret.)
Uniformed Services University of the Health Sciences
Bethesda, MD

JEFF T. DYAR, NREMT-P
National Fire Academy, Federal Emergency Management Agency
Emmitsburg, MD

Maj. BRIAN ZACHARIAH, MD, FACEP, USAR
University of Texas Southwestern Medical Center
Dallas, TX

Sgt. 1st Class ROGER HILLHOUSE, RRT, CVT, EMT
US Army Medical Department Center and School
Ft. Sam Houston, TX

HENRY J. SIEGELSON, MD, FACEP
Emory University
Atlanta, GA

LTC CLIFF CLOONAN, MD, FACEP
Joint Special Operations Medical Training Center
Ft. Bragg, NC

JONATHAN F. POLITIS, REMT-P
Emergency Medical Services
Colonie, NY

Maj. PETER FORSBERG, MA, PA-C, US Army (Ret)
University of Texas Health Science Center
San Antonio, TX

Mstr. Chief LOUIS P. BROCKETT, NREMT, IDC
Naval Hospital
Patuxent River, MD

Sgt. Maj. BRADLEY ENNIS

US Army Medical Command
Ft. Sam Houston, TX

JOSHUA VAYER, EMT-P
Casualty Care Research Center
Bethesda, MD

Capt. ERIC M. JOHNSON, RN, NREMT
US Army Medical Department Center and School
Ft. Sam Houston, TX

CMSgt ROBERT LOFTUS, EMT, USAF
Command Medical Service Manager
Langley Air Force Base, VA

ERIC POACH, EMT-P
EMS Outreach Specialist
Mercy Hospital of Pittsburg, PA

MSgt RICHARD ELLIS, NREMT-P, USAF
USAF EMT Program Manager
Wichita Falls, TX

JAMES JONES, Director of Emergency Preparedness

Niagara Mohawk Corp. Nuclear Power Plant
Oswego, NY

Ptl. JAMES S. HOLMAN, EMT-P
Alleghany County Bureau of Police, SWAT
Pittsburgh, PA

ANDREW DORMAN, Supervisory Special Agent
Federal Bureau of Investigation, Bomb Data Center
Washington, DC

CHRIS THOMPSON, EMT-P, USN (Ret)
Rural Metro Ambulance Service
Syracuse, NY

Staff Sgt. EVERETT TAYLOR, CVT
Brooke Army Medical Center
Ft. Sam Houston, TX

Sgt. 1st Class STEVEN NEWSOME, EMT, CVT
US Army Medical Department Center and School
Ft. Sam Houston, TX

1

MEDICAL ASPECTS OF WMD

INTRODUCTION

Terrorism is an unfortunate reality of modern society. The Oklahoma City bombing in 1995 (Figure 1-1) and sarin nerve agent attack in Tokyo in 1996 have driven the need to plan and prepare for terrorism. This handbook is designed to address the medical effects of terrorist attacks. The focus will be the assessment and management of patients in the prehospital arena. Additional information on decontamination, disaster preparedness and mass casualty management will also be outlined. The goal is to give the prehospital provider the information needed to successfully handle casualties from terrorist weapons.

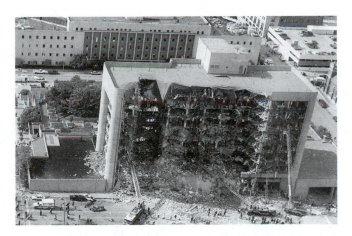

Figure 1-1 The scene of the Oklahoma City federal building bombing April 19, 1995.

By choice, terrorists frequently employ weapons of mass destruction. By definition, these weapons cause widespread, indiscriminate death and destruction. Nuclear, biologic and chemical weapons are the most likely weapons of mass destruction (WMD). Conventional explosives are now also considered to be WMD. Under certain circumstances the destructive power of conventional bombs can be sufficient to cause great damage. This was evident in Oklahoma City and at the World Trade Center (Figure 1-2). Furthermore, the historical importance of terrorist bombs and the relative availability of explosives demands a discussion of this weapon. Incendiary devices will also be included.

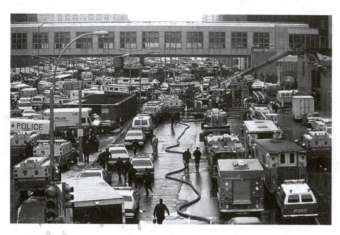

Figure 1-2 The scene of the World Trade Center bombing, February 26, 1993.

Destructive Power

WMD have the potential for widespread and devastating destruction. Just a few ounces of chemical agent can kill hundreds of people. Some biologic agents are even more potent. It is possible to fit a small nuclear weapon in a footlocker with the power to completely obliterate at least 10 city blocks and damage many more. In contrast, the Oklahoma City bomb fit inside a truck and destroyed the equivalent of one city block. Table 1-1 illustrates the comparative power of the major weapons of mass destruction.

The potential to cause physical destruction and death varies with each type of WMD. Conventional explosives can cause serious damage to a limited area, but rarely affect more than a city block or two. Nuclear bombs can cause utter destruction of property and very high death and injury rates in the area of the blast. Chemical weapons, at least in theory, can kill even more people because a small amount of agent can be spread over a wide area such as a densely populated metropolitan area. Physical destruction of property is minimal but environmental contamination can be serious and prolonged.

TABLE 1-1

LIKELIHOOD OF RISK AND POTENTIAL OVERALL DESTRUCTIVE POWER OF WEAPONS OF MASS DESTRUCTION

WEAPON	LIKELIHOOD	DESTRUCTIVE POWER
conventional explosives	highest	lowest
chemical agent	moderate	moderate
biologic agents	moderate	moderate–high
nuclear weapons	lowest	highest

Biological weapons, because of their insidious nature and ability to spread through contagion, can potentially cause huge numbers of deaths. Table 1-2 provides a perspective on the comparative lethality of the most worrisome forms of WMD.

Onset of Action

Nuclear and conventional bombs have obvious, immediate effects (nuclear weapons may have delayed effects, too.) Chemical and biologic agents may be more insidious. Additionally, the time, course or duration of effects ranges from immediate to days and weeks. Table 1-3 provides illustrative comparisons of these effects.

TABLE 1-2

COMPARATIVE DESTRUCTIVE POWER OF 50 KG OF A HIGHLY EFFECTIVE WMD, DEPLOYED AGAINST A CITY OF 500,000

WEAPON	KILLED	INFRASTRUCTURE DAMAGE	ENVIRONMENTAL CONTAMINATION
Nuclear	100,000	High	High
Chemical	150,000	Minimal	High
Biological	200,000	Minimal	Minimal

TABLE 1-3

COMPARATIVE ONSET AND DURATION OF WMD

WEAPON	ONSET	DURATION
Conventional Explosive	Immediate	Momentary
Nuclear	Immediate	Momentary (fallout: Days-Weeks)
Chemical	Minutes	Minutes-Hours
Biological	Hours-Days	Days-Weeks

Risk

Weapons of mass destruction range from simple mixtures of common chemicals to highly complex nuclear fission bombs. Each requires a different approach to acquisition, development and employment to be effective. Table 1-1 describes the general risk or likelihood of use and potential destructive power. By far, conventional explosives represent the greatest risk, and history bears this out. Virtually all major terrorist attacks to date have involved explosives. Fortunately, conventional explosives have limited power to produce mass destruction. Chemical weapons are relatively cheap and easy to produce and may represent the greatest overall risk from a WMD. Some characteristics of chemical agents are shown in Table 1-4. Biologic weapons have tremendous potential to cause widespread deaths and are relatively inexpensive to produce. A few characteristics of biological agents are shown in Table 1-5. Challenges to effectively delivering biologic agents may limit the threat, however. Nuclear weapons can be devastating because of the utter destruction they produce. Some of the characteristics of nuclear weapons are shown in Table 1-6. However, fission bombs are technically difficult to manufacture and maintain, and this limits the likelihood of their use.

Detection

Chemical and biologic agents, and the radiation effects of nuclear weapons are colorless and odorless as a rule. They cannot be detected by human senses until clinical effects have occurred. This has obvious implications in terms of identifying the agent (discussed later). It also makes these weapons insidious in their employment. In contrast, the blast of conventional or nuclear bombs is obvious.

It is also possible for a terrorist to combine various WMD to produce multiple effects. Combining a conventional explosive with a radioactive (but not fissionable)

TABLE 1-4

SOME CHARACTERISTICS OF CHEMICAL AGENTS (AEROSOL DEPLOYMENT)

AGENT	PERSISTENCE		RATE OF ACTION	PORTAL OF ENTRY
	WARM WEATHER	COLD WEATHER		
Nerve				
GA,GB,GD	10 min-24h	2h-3d	very rapid	lungs, eyes
VX	2d-1wk	2d-weeks	rapid	lungs, eyes
Pulmonary				
CG,DP	1m-10m	10m-1h	immediate	lungs, eyes
Vesicant				
HD,HN	3d-1wk	weeks	slow	eyes, skin
L,HL	1d-3d	weeks	rapid	eyes, skin
CX	days	days	very rapid	eyes, skin
Cyanogens				
AC,CK	1m-10m	10m-1h	immediate	lungs

TABLE 1-5

SOME CHARACTERISTICS OF BIOLOGICAL AGENTS (AEROSOL DEPLOYMENT)

AGENT	STABILITY	INCUBATION TIME	LETHALITY
Anthrax	high	1d-6d	high
Botulinum	high	24h-36h	high
Cholera	moderate	1d-5d	moderate
Plague	low	2wks-3wks	moderate
Ricin	high	12h-36h	high
Staphylococcus Enterotoxin B	high	1h-6h	low
Trichothecene Mycotoxin T4	high	minutes-hours	moderate
Tularemia	low	2d-10d	moderate

material produces a weapon with the capacity to spread radioactive material over a wide area. Chemical or biological agents can similarly be combined with conventional explosives.

The goal of a terrorist attack, in simple terms, is to frighten (terrorize) or coerce the public and WMD are certainly effective in this regard. The prehospital implications of this terror potential are enormous. Public panic, mass hysteria, overload of communications systems and clogging of the highways will add to the misery of the actual disaster effects. Chapter 2, Prehospital Response will discuss some of these implications.

PREHOSPITAL APPROACH

The general prehospital approach to dealing with WMD is similar to that of any disaster. The principles of disaster response remain the same, with a few additions. Local, regional and state disaster plans should consider the possibility of WMD attacks. Table 1-7 lists several important considerations to consider in responses to WMD disasters.

TABLE 1-6

SOME DESTRUCTIVE CHARACTERISTICS OF NUCLEAR WEAPONS (AIRBURST)

| SIZE | RANGE OF EFFECTS (DIAMETER IN KM) | | | |
	LETHAL RADIATION	LETHAL BLAST	SERIOUS MISSILE INJURY	SERIOUS BURNS
1 kT	0.7	0.3	0.2	0.8
20 kT	1.3	1.0	0.6	1.8
100 kT	1.6	1.4	1.5	3.2
1 MT	2.3	3.8	3.6	4.8
10 MT	3.7	11.7	NA	14.5

NA=Not available

TABLE 1-7

CONSIDERATIONS IN THE APPROACH TO WMD RESPONSE

Personal & public safety is paramount.
Contain the hazard and control access.
Implement appropriate ICS response.
Triage and treat casualties.
Protect the crime scene.

Safety

The biggest concern when responding to a terrorist attack is to assure the safety of the response team and the public. All WMD attacks have the potential for contaminating large areas. Proper protective equipment and devices are needed to safely operate in contaminated areas (Figure 1-3). A further risk is additional or secondary devices designed to injure or kill the rescuers. Proper training and strict adherence to safety procedures will minimize the risk to responders. An effective public evacuation plan will mitigate the risk to the public.

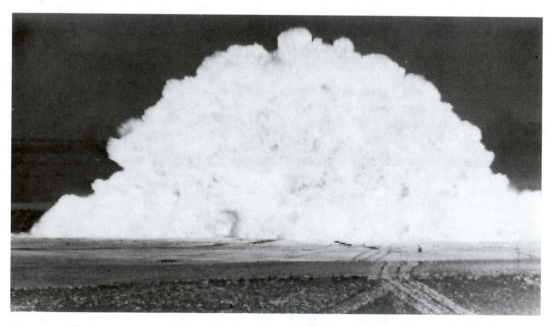

Figure 1-3 The WMD scene can pose significant hazards to resources. Here, a powerful conventional explosive is tested in the southwestern desert.

Containment

Minimizing the spread of chemical, biological or radioactive contamination will minimize additional casualties and reduce future clean-up costs. Hazardous materials (hazmat) teams are familiar with containment procedures and must be an integral part of any WMD response.

Containment also means patient decontamination (Figure 1-4). All victims of a WMD should have all their clothes removed (see section on protecting the crime scene in this chapter for care of clothing articles) before any transportation. Appropriate decontamination must follow before the patient is moved to the hospital. Chapter 4, Care of Chemical Injuries, and Chapter 7, Personal Protection and Patient Decontamination, provide additional details on these procedures

Psychological Effects

Undoubtedly, a WMD will cause widespread death and destruction. In addition to the physical effects of the weapon (blast, shrapnel, radiation, contamination of the community, etc.), significant psychological effects can be expected. Survivors will show varying degrees of stress reaction to the disaster. This can be independent of or in combination with physical effects. Prehospital providers will need to prepare for the possibility of hundreds or thousands of patients needing psychological support. Special multidisciplinary teams of physicians, psychologists, social workers, chaplains, and other mental health specialists may be needed after a WMD attack.

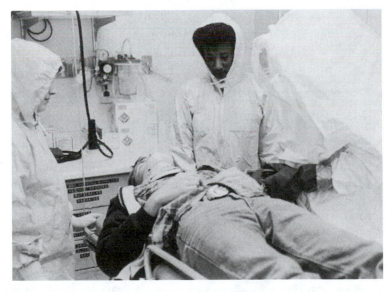

Figure 1-4 Patient decontamination requires special training and equipment.

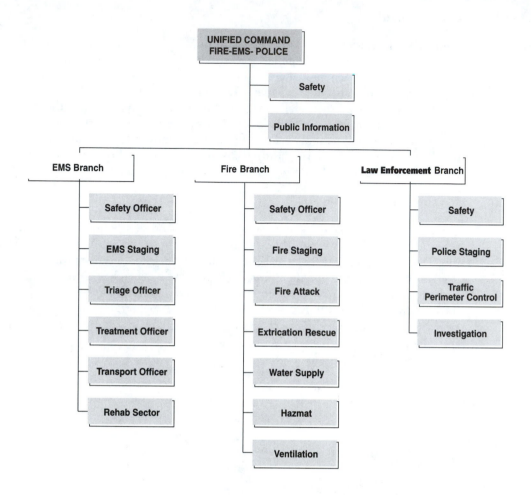

Figure 1-5 Incident Command System organization.

Rescue and healthcare personnel are not immune to psychological stress. Critical incident stress debriefing (CISD) protocols have been developed to mitigate psychological trauma. While not proven to reduce the long term effects of psychological trauma, CISD offers people an opportunity to relieve stress and feel better and remains an important element of post-incident management.

Triage

The medical effects of WMD are varied and range from mild to severe. By their very nature, WMD will cause hundreds, perhaps thousands of casualties. Triage, or medical sorting can be critically important in the emergency care of a WMD incident. Therefore all prehospital providers should be as comfortable with mass casualty triage as they are with the individual treatment of WMD casualties.

Disaster Response

The major thrust of the response to terrorist WMD is the disaster response. It is beyond the scope of this handbook to detail all the elements and principles of planning a disaster response. Chapter 2, Prehospital Response, outlines the basics. Interested readers are invited to review any of the fine textbooks on disaster medicine for additional information.

The first step in the disaster response should be to activate the local disaster plan and initiate the incident command system (ICS) (Figure 1-5). ICS is a method of command, control and organization for major incident responses. It uses standardized elements and procedures to allow agencies from many different locations to work together. All prehospital providers should understand their role in the local ICS plan.

Protect the Crime Scene

Terrorist attacks are crime scenes as well as medical or disaster scenes. Police and other law enforcement officials have primary responsibility in securing the scene and collecting criminal evidence. In the US, the Federal Bureau of Investigation (FBI) will likely have jurisdiction in the event of a WMD release. Prehospital providers share in this responsibility to protect evidence. Table 1-8 provides several considerations. Save all potential evidence, even if seemingly trivial. Place all clothing and personal articles in a paper bag (paper prevents rapid molding and decay of organic evidence). Place the paper bag in an airtight plastic bag, then rebag again with airtight plastic. Label each bag appropriately, and control the storage of the evidence. Bagging in this fashion both preserves the evidence and helps minimize the spread of contamination. And lastly, be sure to document carefully, as the written record may later be entered as evidence.

Community Effects

By their very nature, WMD will cause widespread effects to the local community. Disruption of many or all infrastructures will hamper the medical response. Hospitals, fire and EMS stations, communications centers and other vital facilities may be damaged, destroyed or inaccessible. Roads, airports, and transportation control systems may fail. Communication may be difficult or impossible. Vehicles and equipment may be

TABLE 1-8

CONSIDERATIONS IN PROTECTING THE CRIME SCENE

Place clothing and personal articles in paper bags
Place paper bags in double plastic bags
Cut clothing around, not through shrapnel holes
Save all evidence and document clearly

inoperative or contaminated. Available rescue personnel may be injured, ill or unable to reach the scene. In summary, a disaster has occurred. This must all be considered and planned for in a WMD response.

For purposes of this handbook, we will assume the WMD has affected a large part of a given community, but has not totally obliterated the community disaster response. Massive disasters such as strategic or regional thermonuclear war are of such proportions that meaningful medical response is unlikely, and therefore will not be directly addressed in this handbook.

SUMMARY

Weapons of mass destruction are among the most frightening of all disasters. They can be both insidious and hideous in their effects. With proper training and preparation, pre-hospital providers can, however, prepare for the medical effects.

FOR FURTHER READING

Emergency Response to Terrorism: Basic Concepts Student Manual. US Fire Administration, National Fire Academy. Emmitsburg, MD, 1997

DANON YL, et al (eds): Chemical Warfare Medicine. Gefen Publishing House, Ltd. Jerusalem, 1994.

SPIERS EM: Chemical and Biological Weapons. St. Martin's Press. New York, 1984

ZAJTCHUK R, et al (eds): Medical Aspects of Chemical and Biological Warfare. Department of the Army, Office of the Surgeon General, Washington, DC, 1997

HOLLOWAY HC, et al: The threat of biological weapons. JAMA 1997; 278: 425-427 Christopher GW, et al: Biological warfare: A historical perspective. JAMA 1997; 278: 412-417

Textbook of Military Medicine (Part 1, Volume 2) Medical Consequences of Nuclear Warfare. Office of the Surgeon General, Washington, D.C. 1990

Manual of Protective Action Guidelines and Protective Action for Nuclear Incidents: Environmental Protection Agency, Washington, D.C. 1992 (EPA-400-R-92-001)

GRACE, C.: Nuclear Weapons: Principles, Effects and Survivability, Brassey's Limited, London, UK. 1995

CHRISTEN, H., MANISCALCO, P.: The EMS Incident Management System: EMS Operations for Mass Casualty and High Impact Incidents. Prentice-Hall, Upper Saddle River, NJ 1998.

AUF DER HEIDE, E.: Disaster Response: Principles of Preparation and Coordination. C. V. Mosby Company, St. Louis, MO. 1989

Health Service Support in a Nuclear, Biological, and Chemical Environment, Field Manual 8-10-7. Department of the Army, Washington, DC, 1993.

2

PREHOSPITAL RESPONSE

INTRODUCTION

The current state of society and technology makes incidents like the Oklahoma City Federal Building bombing and the Tokyo Subway nerve agent attack more likely throughout the world and here at home. Our role in the face of this threat is to plan and prepare for the event, respond safely, and to be able to provide the needed triage, decontamination, assessment, care, and transport. Post incident, this role also entails clean-up, providing an incident review, and preparation for another response.

As this text presents, there are basically five forms of mass destruction weapons: biological contamination, nuclear detonation, incendiary fires, toxic chemical release, and conventional explosion (B NICE). Each of these potential disasters requires an EMS response different from the normal or even extreme situations to which you are accustomed. The scale and scope of death and destruction, the insidious nature of the weapon, and the personal danger to care-givers all make these incidents of special concern.

Without planning for such an incident, we risk being ill-prepared to provide the best support and care to those injured and may also risk our lives unnecessarily. Such an event may have a great psychological impact on us as care providers unless we are ready to deal with the degree of destruction and injury and are counseled and supported thereafter.

PLANNING AND PREPARATION FOR WEAPONS OF MASS DESTRUCTION

Weapons of mass destruction are able to kill and maim thousands in very short periods of time. A 20 megaton nuclear detonation will kill 50% of personnel at 10 miles from the blast from burns alone, and accomplishes an increasing mortality as you approach ground zero. Chemical weapons may kill all those in a one to twenty-block area almost immediately, while biological weapons may kill hundreds or thousands days or weeks after an unrealized exposure. These extremely devastating events can, without warning, take you from the everyday nature of EMS activity to a prolonged and desperate encounter. If you are to do the most good for the greatest number and ultimately accomplish the highest survival, you must prepare operationally, physically, and mentally for the event.

In planning for the WMD incident, consider several aspects of preparation and response. The scope of these disasters quickly exhausts resources and their nature may require massive quantities of supplies not normally available in large numbers. These incidents require special protective gear that must be available in very large quantities to support extrication, triage, decontamination, and clean-up. Transportation resources to distribute casualties well beyond the normal patient flow patterns are needed, as are personnel to drive or fly them and to provide medical support and limited care en route. Communications may be totally disrupted with a nuclear detonation or by terrorist actions in support of a WMD attack. And, with the nuclear detonation, the local or regional civilian and medical care infrastructure may be severely disrupted or destroyed. These factors make planning for the terrorist weapon of mass destruction critical if you and the EMS system are to respond adequately and safely.

Supply and Equipment Inventory

Planning for a weapon of mass destruction release requires an inventory of equipment and supplies in the community. It is unrealistic to expect that when the incident occurs your system will then be able to search out where particular materials are found and rapidly access them. As described in the next few chapters of this text, each type of WMD incident requires certain necessary medications and medical equipment for an appropriate response. For example, a nerve agent release requires massive amounts of atropine and the use of large numbers of ventilators. A community inventory of these items, and more importantly, a listing of places that have large supplies, like pharmaceutical warehouses, medical supply houses, and home care agencies, is essential. This inventory may not only help your community respond to a local incident but may help in response to an incident in a neighboring community.

The WMD response also requires access to specially trained personnel and response equipment. Entry into a chemical release may require SCBA, Hazmat, or NBC protection as well as personnel practiced in their use. A large explosion and associated structural collapse may call for heavy equipment, search and rescue teams, special electronic equipment, or specially trained dogs. The dispatch center must have a method of quickly accessing these resources in great numbers. This need may require a regional, statewide, or nationwide response.

Medical Direction

Beyond the medical equipment and supplies and specialty personnel, it is important to plan for the intense EMS operations needed during a weapon of mass destruction incident. There will be large numbers of care providers, including some from regions with different medical control systems and protocols. Your EMS system must plan how these providers are to receive medical direction. With the expected communications system overload, consider taking emergency measures to have all protocols as standing orders with only special circumstances calling for online medical direction. This assures that communication channels are available for scene updates, incoming patient reports, and only those care provider-physician communications essential to acute patient care. It is important that direct online medical control be available when a care provider is presented with a special or extraordinary circumstance, like a patient trapped and in need of possible field amputation.

Your system must also develop special protocols for specific WMD incidents. An example might include appropriate atropine dosages for nerve agents. Special protocols must also address patient flow. They should direct minor injuries and walking wounded away from the hospitals nearest the incident to permit hospitals to extend greater resources to the seriously affected casualties.

Provider Preparation

It is also important that individual providers are aware of the personal risks and dangers associated with a weapon of mass destruction response. Walking into a sarin nerve agent cloud could mean immediate death or permanent disability to a provider who does not respect the real dangers of this threat. Responding to a biological threat may appear like a flu outbreak and lead to a delayed and agonizing responder illness or death. Rushing into the scene of an explosion to provide immediate care may result in rescuer deaths, a second objective of terrorist attacks. A true respect for the insidious nature of secondary devices and their users is essential to safeguard those who respond to WMD incidents. This respect comes from a clear understanding of the terrorist's intentions and the nature of the devices they are now using.

As an EMS provider, you need to be aware of the special treatment and transport protocols a WMD incident requires. You must have immediate access to written protocols (for review and direction at the time of the incident) addressing each type of agent: biological, nuclear, incendiary, chemical, and explosive (B NICE). These protocols must identify the specific signs and symptoms caused by the agent and the recommended treatments. You must further have guidance in recognizing the effects of the various agents, then triage patients into expectant, immediate, delayed, and ambulatory categories for care and transport. Your safety requires you to be aware of the dangers each agent presents to your health and what precautions are required before entering the scene, during care, and after the response.

Response-Provider Logistics

Your pre-planning must also consider the massive and prolonged response the WMD incident requires. There will likely be more responders on scene than for any previous system response, and they will be there for many hours, possibly days. To assist their efforts, response support needs to provide meals, hot or cold fluids, frequent rest and sleep periods, bathroom facilities, and medical care for these providers. In your plan, identify where and from whom these materials will come and who will support and coordinates this aspect of the response effort. It is also advisable to staff heavy work areas with care provider shifts so relief is regular.

Incident Command System

The weapon of mass destruction incident is similar to a large-scale natural disaster. Here, as with any serous disaster, the incident requires a system to provide overall emergency services coordination. The **incident command system**, as discussed in most EMS and fire service textbooks, is the most practical model for response control and coordination (Figure2-1). One individual is identified as the incident commander, usually from the fire service, and he or she works from one location with distinct command chains for each discipline and strategic area involved in the response. Resources are coordinated through the command structure and sectors are established for each major task and staging of the operation. For emergency medical service, the major sectors are triage, treatment, and transport. Very large incidents require numerous sub-command locations to oversee geographic

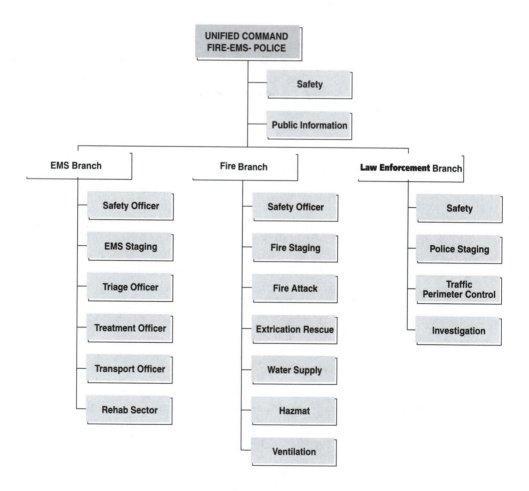

Figure 2-1   Incident command system organization.

sub-areas of the incident. For example, a nuclear detonation will likely have many incident command areas, coordinated by a central command. Communication occurs with a central overall command to assure a coordinated allocation of supplies, equipment and personnel.

The WMD incident may also require special sectors affecting EMS. For example, in the chemical exposure, there is the need for a victim removal or extrication sector. Here fire service or Hazmat personnel with SCBA, Hazmat, or NBC equipment remove victims from the hazardous exposure and to a safe triage sector. In the biological or nuclear weapon release, a decontamination sector may be essential to remove the hazard before you can safely provide any care or transport.

Security and Safety

Unlike normal EMS responses, those responsible for the terrorist incident may wish to limit or sabotage your ability to respond. Hospitals should establish and maintain security perimeters and limit access to facilities to only those with need and authorization for entry. EMS and scene personnel must have easily recognizable photo type identification to discourage unauthorized personnel from infiltrating the system. Your system also must appreciate that terrorists, determined to disrupt the system and with the advantage of their own preplanning, may be very effective at interfering with our ability to respond, communicate, and function effectively. Be particularly wary of secondary devices (e.g., bombs) deployed in such a manner as to kill or injure rescuers.

The police (and possibly active and reserve military units) should know the structure of the typical response, the command structure, the personnel involved, and the accepted forms of authorized personnel identification. In fact, all units and agencies anticipating a response or support function to a WMD incident should be familiar with and be prepared to operate under the ICS.

Psychological Preparation

Personally, you need to be ready to deal with the nature and scope of a disaster and that someone intentionally caused the conflagration. Recognize that you, who are here to alleviate death and suffering can be emotionally devastated by intentional acts that cause injury and death, especially with nature and magnitude of a weapon of mass destruction. These events are likely in modern society and your role is to intervene aggressively to salvage those that can be saved. While massive death and severe and devastating injury are difficult for anyone to handle, it is important that you recognize the reality of these incidents, yet remain effective in light of the human suffering they present. Then go on with your life, hopefully, without serious psychological scars.

Interagency Coordination

Planning for a WMD incident must also consider the working relationships of the various agencies involved in the response. Before the call for such a response, fire, EMS, police, and other support services must define their respective roles and responsibilities at the scene. This includes all levels of governmental response from local, regional and state to federal levels. This information must be common knowledge to the leadership of each service and shared with individual responders to limit scene confusion. Since the incident's magnitude will likely be great and services and personnel will be drawn from surrounding communities, regional pre-planning, coordination, and rehearsal is essential. Should communications be compromised, this readiness will support a coordinated and efficient response.

RESPONDING TO WEAPON OF MASS DESTRUCTION INCIDENTS

One of the most crucial aspects of WMD incident deployment is recognition. Your EMS community must appreciate that these incidents are becoming more and more likely. Preparation and anticipation are the only ways to protect yourself and fellow rescuers and assure an effective response when the terrorist employs a weapon of mass destruction. The earlier you recognize what is happening, the earlier you can protect yourself and access outside resources necessary for an effective response.

Conventional or nuclear detonations are over when you are aware of what has happened. However, with a terrorist bombing, be wary of a secondary device or booby traps designed to endanger you and fellow rescuers. Be prepared for these detonation hazards to assure your safety and those of other rescuers.

There is a significant difference between the effects of conventional, chemical, and (most) biological weapons and the death, injury, and mass destruction of the nuclear weapon. The former accounts for a relatively small region of impact and places extreme strain on the EMS system and medical care, yet the system infrastructure (facilities and personnel) remains largely intact. A large nuclear weapon, on the other hand, creates concentric rings of complete destruction, severe devastation, and areas of limited damage, superimposed upon the death and injury. This physical destruction severely limits access to the immense scene and destroys all the response and health care components within its rings. Gone too are the shelters, medical and food supplies, and available clean water. Nuclear devices may also destroy electrical equipment quite remote from the epicenter, including radios and computers. This may leave the entire response without effective communications and operable dispatch centers. Then there is the eminent danger from fallout that begins about one hour after the detonation and continues for days and weeks. The response to a sizable nuclear event will require extreme measures to evacuate, care for, and support the injured.

Chemical and biological weapons present a danger that is much more difficult to identify than the conventional or nuclear detonation. Chemical weapons may release gases or aerosols that are only recognized upon exposure or shortly thereafter. When reports of "numerous ill patients from an unidentifiable cause" are received, anticipate a threatening environment until proven otherwise. Often the casualties will complain of respiratory symptoms like cough, a "burning chest and eyes," and difficulty breathing. Excessive salivation, loss of bowel and bladder control, and tearing may indicate danger. Dead animals and insects or those in a state of incapacitation may suggest a chemical exposure. Odors of bitter almonds, peaches, mustard, or fresh cut grass may also be indicators of deadly gases.

With biological weapons, exposure occurs well before the first signs and symptoms appear. It may be hard to determine the exact agent and contamination source for hours or days. The biological release may also affect the entire EMS and emergency medical infrastructure before the problem's nature is known. Smallpox, for example, may leave its first victims ill, entering the medical system, and spreading the virus well before a diagnosis is made. By the time someone recognizes the incident nature, most care givers will be exposed. Then there is little that can be done. However, when you are presented with signs and symptoms of a community disease, take body substance isolation precautions. Employ HEPA mask, gloves, and gowns for personal protection, and alert medical control. It is possible that many large city EMS responders will be inoculated against the major biological threats in the next few years.

The direction of your approach to a suspected chemical, nuclear, or biological weapon deployment is crucial. Ideally access the scene from upwind. If the area is exceptionally large or entry is limited, the next best approach is from the side. Avoid accessing the scene from downwind and be wary of shifting wind during the response. Be cautious of confined spaces like subways, basement areas, the confines of large buildings or low lying geographical areas. These areas may contain the chemical or biological agent and remain unsafe for unprotected entry until adequately ventilated.

The target of a terrorist act is often something that is either used heavily by or greatly impacts the population. Such locations might be airports, subways, schools, churches, government buildings or large public gatherings such as fairs or festivals. Whenever you are called to these locations, anticipate a possible terrorist act.

When suspicious of a WMD incident, remain remote from the scene until you can ascertain the incident's nature and take the proper personal protective actions. Once an incident is recognized, immediately employ the incident command structure and do a careful scene size-up to begin a coordinated, organized, and effective response. It is also important to immediately establish a perimeter for the safety of fellow rescuers and the public.

Your Role at the WMD Incident

The WMD incident requires one of three roles for you as an EMS provider. If you arrive as the first unit in, establish incident command, do a quick scene size-up, and communicate essential information to the dispatch center. If you are among the first EMS providers in or play an EMS system leadership role, provide or help provide sector leadership. Otherwise, go about rendering assessment and triage (in the triage sector), care (in the treatment sector), packaging and patient loading (in the transport sector) or possibly some care while transporting numerous casualties via ambulance or other vehicle to a nearby or remote care facility. Figure 2-2 outlines your initial role on the scene of a WMD/hazardous material mass casualty incident.

Incident Command

As the first or one of the first units to arrive at a WMD incident, perform the scene size-up. Resist the urge to provide care to those who present as needing it immediately. The size-up identifies the incident's nature and scope and will set the stage for the entire response. The information you gather and communicate to dispatch determines the speed and appropriateness of your system's response. It may very well be the most important few minutes of the disaster response.

EMT RESPONSIBILITIES AT A HAZMAT INCIDENT

Recognize and report the hazmat incident.

▼

Establish control of the scene.

▼

Identify the substance involved. Use, as appropriate, these resources:
- NFPA 704 System
- U.S. DOT labels and placards
- Interviews with people on scene
- Shipping documents
- Material Safety Data Sheets
- *North American Emergency Response Guidebook*
- CHEMTREC
- CHEMTEL, Inc.
- Poison Control centers

▼

Establish a medical treatment site.

▼

Perform rehabilitation operations.

▼

Care for the injured.

INITIAL EMT RESPONSIBILITIES AT AN MCI

First arriving EMTs establish EMS Command. Put on proper identification.

▼

Walk through the scene (or observe from a safe distance for a hazmat incident). Assess for:
- Number of patients
- Scene hazards
- Apparent patient priorities
- Need for extrication
- Number of ambulances needed
- Other factors affecting the scene
- Resources needed to address them
- Areas in which to stage resources

▼

Radio in an initial scene report with request for additional resources.

▼

Organize, deciding where to place resources and what sectors will be needed. Sectors may include the following:
- Staging
- Supply
- Extrication
- Triage
- Treatment
- Transportation
- Rehab

▼

Begin initial triage of patients if appropriate.

▼

Assign incoming units and personnel to appropriate sectors.

Figure 2-2   Initial roles of the EMS provider at a WMD/hazardous materials mass casualty incident.

Identify a location for incident command that has a reasonable view of the scene. This permits you to identify essential geographic locations for sectors and direct units in and out. Communicate this location to dispatch as they will direct incoming service leadership to this site for assignment. Dispatch will assign a radio frequency for incident command to assure you good communications with the various responding disciplines.

Determine the incident nature. Is it a chemical exposure, a biological agent release, or an explosion? Determine how it effects the casualties. Are they severely debilitated or do they have only minor complaints or injuries? What is the scope of the incident? Are dozens, hundreds or thousands ill or hurt? What are the geographic bounds? Is it one building, a block, or an entire neighborhood? Do all you can to accurately describe what is going on well enough for dispatch and the EMS system to begin an appropriate response.

View the disaster area to determine routes of egress for other responding units, areas for their staging, areas for triage and treatment of patients, and routes for travel away from the scene by units transporting patients. We have learned from incidents like the Bianca airplane crash on Long Island that some initial thought to vehicle placement and flow at the beginning of an incident pays off well as the incident progresses. Again, communicate this information to dispatch and begin establishing sectors as early as you can.

Consider the essential services required for this incident. Determine where each sector is best located and the requirements for proper performance. Assure reasonable traffic patterns for units and personnel moving into and out of the scene to limit congestion. Assign geographic space for extrication, triage, decontamination, assessment, and care sectors as needed. Select areas that are free of danger and can be secured against bystander or possible terrorist infiltration. As fire, police and EMS units arrive, assign officers as appropriate to coordinate the activities at each sector.

Once ranking emergency service personnel arrive at the scene, provide them with a complete briefing on what you have found and what sectors and areas you have established. As they feel comfortable with the information and scene management, relinquish your command responsibilities and assume more normal EMS provider activity. You will likely provide sector management or care in a specific sector. The likely EMS sectors at a WMD incident include triage, treatment, and transport, and possibly extrication and decontamination.

Triage

In true disaster situations, where the casualties far outstrip the available resources, employ the START (Simple Triage And Rapid Treatment) system of triage (Figure 2-3). Here you will call for casualties to extract themselves from danger. This moves casualties quickly from further contamination and injury and triages the least injured away from the incident. There may be merit to move these first evacuees via bus or truck to remote health care facilities. Otherwise, their likely minor or moderate injuries and their sheer numbers will add to the care system overload. Also, consider the use of other than normal emergency patient destinations like health care clinics, physician offices, or walk-in and urgent care centers.

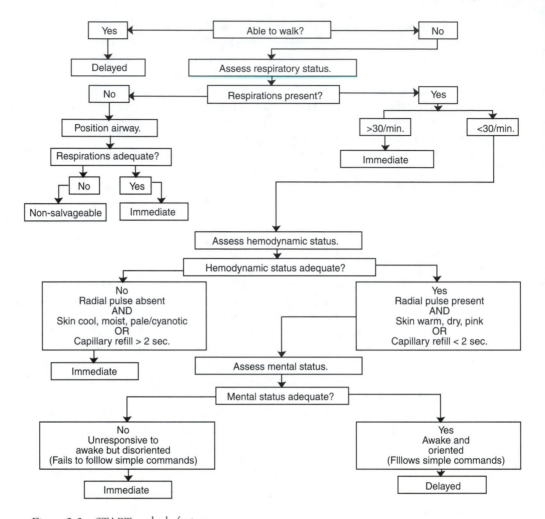

Figure 2-3 START method of triage.

Once minor casualties are extracted from the scene, divide those remaining into serious but salvageable and those who are in cardiac arrest. In an incident of disaster scope, resources are not available to resuscitate the pulseless patient. Determine casualties who are alive but with apparent mortal injuries. They must be left without care and quickly made comfortable (expectant). Devoting resources to them leaves other more easily stabilized casualties without care. Care for casualties with serious but salvageable injuries first (immediate), followed by those classified as delayed and ambulatory.

The military has successfully employed a system of triage that at times cares for the least injured first and works toward the most severely injured. In battle conditions this conserves the fighting force and directs the greatest resources to those who can return to fight. In the major disaster, by the time the emergency response gets under full steam, many seriously and mortally injured or affected victims will have already died. In these dire circumstances it may be reasonable to provide early care to those capable of rapidly contributing to the relief effort. This will most likely mean treating and returning to duty fellow rescuers who are injured at the scene.

Triage may expose you to the deadly agent responsible for the incident. Hence, it may be essential to perform your tasks while dressed in NBC or hazmat gear. You are generally warmer and activity is more restricted and exhausting in the suit. You will require frequent rest periods and greater fluid intake. It is advisable that you practice providing care while in these suits before asked to do so at a WMD incident.

Treatment

A major activity of EMS at the WMD scene is to provide onscene treatment in anticipation of casualty transport to medical facilities. Here again your responsibilities greatly differ from the normal EMS response or even the multi-casualty incident. There are a large number of casualties all suffering from the same or related medical problems or injuries. Massive soft tissue wounds associated with a terrorist blast, burns from a nuclear or incendiary ignition, or medication needs for a chemical exposure quickly outstrip the normal medical supplies for these problems and require careful rationing and some improvisation on your part. Care providers will be in short supply, leaving you with a higher care provider-to-patient ratio than ever experienced in your career. Adequate personnel, supplies, and equipment may not arrive in sufficient quantities until many hours or even days into the incident.

Patient problems may also require care modalities not normally addressed by your protocols (for example, high dose atropine for nerve agents). Another divergence from normal EMS is that casualties may remain at the treatment sector for prolonged periods of time, needing nourishment, hydration, and personal hygiene considerations.

Finally, the responsibility of attending to casualties who are triaged as expectant and expected to die can be frustrating. Normally in EMS you are with casualties for up to an hour but rarely longer. You may watch patients die, but usually from severe injury or a critical medical insult while you offer aggressive care and resuscitation. In the WMD incident you may be with a patient for hours as they move from a serious exposure to agonizing death, slowly before your eyes. Once death has occurred, you must provide for isolation and storage until after living casualties are evacuated. This may require commandeering refrigeration units such as semi-trailers or rail cars.

Transport

The transport sector is a packaging and loading area in preparation of moving casualties away from the scene and toward care facilities. Here the first priority is often to remove the walking wounded by bus or another mass movement vehicle. They need to be moved well away from the immediate vicinity for two reasons. First, their sheer numbers and need for care will overcrowd and overburden local medical facilities. Secondly, they can tolerate the travel time to remote facilities where personnel are able to devote time to their care. This quick removal from the scene reduces congestion and permits triage and treatment of more seriously wounded victims.

The transport sector must also begin transports of seriously affected casualties very early into the incident. Since the number of these patients is very high, early transport draws out their arrival at hospitals over a longer period of time, giving these facilities more time to address casualty injuries. Have the first EMS units quickly offload their care equipment and supplies at the treatment area, and then load multiple patients. Select patients who are in serious condition but require limited en route care.

Arrange traffic flow from the transport sector to distribute casualties between care facilities. This requires an overall coordination between several transport sectors located within the large WMD incident and receiving facilities. Otherwise, some hospitals become inundated with patients while others are under challenged.

Extrication

An extrication sector may exist at the WMD scene. In the explosion, there may be the need to remove casualties from rubble or debris and bring them to a triage and/or treatment area. This may necessitate dedicated personnel and possibly heavy equipment. At the chemical or radiological incident, there may be the need to remove the casualties from the site as the environment might otherwise endanger unprotected care-givers during triage and treatment.

Decontamination

An additional sector staffed by EMS personnel and necessary in some incidents is decontamination. With nuclear, chemical, and some biological agents, casualties need decontamination between the incident and the treatment area. Triage may occur before or after decontamination. Remove clothing, gently rinse the casualty, and wash or clip body hair to remove what agents you can. Then, evaluate the casualty for residual agents so as not to pass them on to other care givers. Contaminated wash water, cleaning materials, and clothing should be isolated for proper disposal.

The Federal Response

In an incident that impacts the medical system beyond its ability to respond, state and federal support is probable. However, these resources will not be available for hours or possibly days, though their contribution may go a long way toward bringing the incident to a close. Individual state responses vary greatly and are beyond this text to detail. The federal response, however, can bring important resources to the scene and remove casualties to remote facilities, thereby relieving the local medical infrastructure.

The Federal Response Program is relatively new and is a consolidation of a number of federal agencies. FEMA (Federal Emergency Management Agency) is the lead and coordinating agency that brings together the departments of defense, health, transportation, and many other federal agencies. This program provides twelve separate functions, numbers 8 and 9 of which involve health and medical services and urban search and rescue. Some states add additional functions to the original 12 (Figure 2-4). The emergency medical response comes in the form of Disaster Medical Assistance Teams (or DMATs). These teams are staffed with 35 medical care providers and are self sufficient for 24 to 72 hours (with resupply carrying them to 10 to 14 days). They usually arrive as soon as 10 to 14 hours after notification and are designed to care for 200 to 250 patients every 24 hours.

The DMAT response may also triage and remove patients from the disaster scene to remote cities prepared to receive and treat WMD casualties. There are around 60 DMAT teams with about 20 in a state of immediate readiness. These teams are intended to integrate with local services and assist with, not assume control of, the incident. They are requested by the state's governor and authorized by the President.

Active military as well as reserve and guard units may provide person power, security, extrication, medical care, and policing actions in support of the disaster response.

ESF	STATE AGENCY	LOCAL AGENCIES
1. Transportation	Dept. of Transportation	Transit Authority, School Board, Council on Aging
2. Communications	Dept. of Management Services	Telephone Company, Emergency Management, Amateur Radio
3. Public Works	Dept. of Transportation	County and Local Public Works, Construction Contractors
4. Firefighting	Dept. of Insurance	Fire/Rescue Dept., Div. of Forestry
5. Information and Planning	Dept. of Community Affairs	Emergency Management, Planning Department
6. Mass Care	American Red Cross	American Red Cross, School Board
7. Resource Support	Dept. of Management Services	Purchasing Dept.
8. Health and Medical	Dept. of Health	Emergency Medical Services, Private Health Agencies, Public Health
9. Search and Rescue	Dept. of Insurance	Fire/Rescue, Volunteer Search Teams, Civil Air Patrol
10. Hazardous Materials	Dept. of Environmental Protection	Emergency Management, Fire/Rescue
11. Food and Water	Dept. of Agriculture and Consumer Affairs	Salvation Army, Agricultural Agent, Red Cross, Water Dept.
12. Energy	Public Service Commission	Power Company, Gas District, Public Works
13. Military Support	Dept. of Military Affairs	Emergency Management
14. Public Information	Dept. of Community Affairs	Emergency Management County and Local PIO
15. Volunteers and Donations	Dept. of Community Affairs	Emergency Management, United Way, Religious Organizations
16. Law Enforcement	Dept. of Law Enforcement	Sheriff's Dept., Local Police

Figure 2-4   Emergency support functions (ESF).

The military is able to respond unlike any other agency, arriving with its own internal command, control, communications, logistics, supplies and transportation. In a large WMD incident, the military will be integral to disaster mitigation, especially clean-up and reconstitution.

Do not expect a substantial federal response early in the event. Federal units are too large and too far away to arrive quickly. Unquestionably, it is the local and regional system's responsibility to plan and prepare for the first 12-48 hours of a WMD response. Help will arrive after that time, but not likely before.

Incident Investigation

The WMD incident may be both a conflagration of injury and despair and a crime scene. Here EMS and the authorities, the police, FBI, and the Department of Energy (DOE) must combine efforts to accomplish patient care, protect the casualties and care providers from further terrorism, and determine what really happened and who caused it. DOE investigates any nuclear detonation or any released radiological contamination, either distributed by a conventional explosion or by other means. The FBI is responsible for investigating terrorist activity and weapon use. These agencies will piece together the weapon delivery system components to determine the device's nature and any details that can identify its maker. They will likely search out all shrapnel and device debris. During your triage and care, attempt to leave the scene as undisturbed as possible. While emergency patient care always takes priority, catching the person responsible for the destruction may prevent future horrors.

Stress Control

The prolonged nature of a WMD response and the toll this takes on care providers can be extreme. We do not normally maintain our response activity for longer than an hour or two. Yet in this very unusual circumstance, we may be caring for acutely injured and dying patients for many hours or days. We need to take frequent rest periods, eat regularly, and drink plenty of fluids. Otherwise our ability to continue care will diminish quickly. The importance of responder wellness at a significant disaster scene merits assigning an individual to oversee this vital service. This monitoring includes awareness of symptoms of extreme stress in the rescuers. Continuous crying, incapacitation, or abnormal behavior may indicate the adverse effects of stress and the need to relieve a rescuer from care responsibilities.

Return to Normal

Once the serious casualties are transported and your responsibilities for care subside, you must begin the clean-up. Here, isolate and dispose of (or set aside for disposal) any contaminated material. Also be sure vehicles are quickly cleaned (or decontaminated as needed), restocked and then staffed with well-rested care providers. Since the incident drains system resources and restocking is a long and labor intensive process, this effort requires energy and coordination. As EMS response units become available, distribute them evenly around the affected area until normal system responses are available.

Personnel Follow-up

Before you release care providers from the scene, evaluate, feed and re-hydrate them, and ensure adequate sleep. It is also important to monitor rescuer activity over the next few days and even months for symptoms of delayed WMD effects or stress syndrome. Watch for abnormal behavior, rage, drinking or drug use, or anti-social behavior. These signs may indicate delayed stress and the need for psychological support. Delayed effects of radiation and chemical and biological agents must always be considered. Symptoms can vary widely and are dependent largely on the type of WMD. The chapter on nuclear, chemical and biologic weapons give specific examples of possible long-term effects and the likely symptoms. To protect rescuers, it is important to keep records of estimated exposures, acute symptoms and treatment received. This medical surveillance is crucial for ensuring peace of mind and effective long-term medical care.

Critical Incident Stress Debriefing (CISD) may possibly help in preventing significant psychological effects from WMD incidents. CISD gives the incident responder an opportunity to identify his or her feelings, to recognize that many responders are likewise impacted by the incident, and to begin the process of accepting the experiences of the disaster response. Simple verbal reassurance, as well as more formalized counseling by chaplains and mental health workers may be just as effective as CISD if employed properly.

Incident Review

After the casualties are transported, clean-up is complete, and after a few days of rest, an incident review is in order. This incident review identifies and focuses on the elements of response that went well. It also identifies those activities that might be improved to more effectively handle any future incident. This information is then passed on to other systems so they have the opportunity to learn from the mistakes. Many of the principles presented in this text were developed from the lessons learned at actual responses.

SUMMARY

Weapons of Mass Destruction wreak havoc upon many more persons than most other events we experience in prehospital emergency care. They are intentional acts designed to kill and maim and in some cases endanger the rescuer. Carefully approach the scene to ensure your safety and quickly determine the nature and scope of the incident. Establish incident command, request equipment, supplies and personnel, and begin to organize the scene. As senior authorities arrive, brief them, relinquish command, and go about serving as a sector officer or care provider in a triage, treatment, or transport sector. At the end of the incident, provide clean-up services and help bring the EMS system back to a state of full readiness for normal EMS responses. Also monitor your peers for the latent effects of stress this incident may cause. Finally, review the incident to identify what response elements worked well and those that could be modified to improve system response. While it is hoped that none of us will respond to a weapon of mass destruction, preparation and planning are essential to provide the best service to those who find themselves in need.

FOR FURTHER READING

AUF DER HEIDE, MD, ERIC, Disaster Response: Principles of Preparation and Coordination, C. V. Mosby Company, St. Louis, MO, USA, 1989.

CRISTEN, HANK, MANISCALCO, PAUL, The EMS Incident Management System, Prentice-Hall, Upper Saddle River, New Jersey, USA, 1998

MITCHELL, JEFF, BRAY, GRADY, Emergency Services Stress: Guidelines for preserving the Health and Careers of Emergency Services Personnel, Prentice-Hall, Upper Saddle River, New Jersey, USA, 1990

BLEDSOE, B. E., PORTER, R.S., SHADE, B. R., Paramedic Emergency Care, 4th Edition, Prentice-Hall, Upper Saddle River, New Jersey, USA, 1997.

Emergency Response to Terrorism, U. S. Department of Justice/Federal Emergency Management Agency, Washington D.C., USA, August 1997.

3

CARE OF EXPLOSIVES AND INCENDIARY INJURIES

INTRODUCTION

This chapter introduces the care of injuries caused by conventional explosives and incendiary devices. Bombs and incendiary devices remain the tools of choice for terrorists. All EMS providers need to be familiar with the effects of these common threats. Knowledge of the care of casualties produced by these weapons is increasingly important in any domestic response to terrorism.

EXPLOSIVES

Explosives function by the extremely rapid (explosive) burning of special fuels. The burning or combustion process occurs so rapidly that the hot gases produced are pushed outward in a violent fashion. The speed or rate of detonation can be as high as 4 miles/s (6,000m/s) for high explosives and 900ft/s (270m/s) for low explosives. This compresses the air surrounding the explosion and forms a shock wave. This shock wave propagates or moves outward at sonic speeds in all directions. This shock wave or blast effect is what causes blast injury

Blast Characteristics

Near the site of the explosion, the shock wave can be very powerful. Blast overpressure is a term used to describe how powerful the shock wave is. Conventional explosives such as trinitrotoluene (TNT) can produce enormous peak overpressures measuring in the thousands of pounds per square inch near the point of detonation (Figure 3-1). Fortunately, this peak overpressure lasts only a few milliseconds and dissipates rapidly with distance. However, even two ounces of TNT can be lethal up to one meter (yard) away. Table 3-1 lists several types of explosives and their power as compared to TNT.

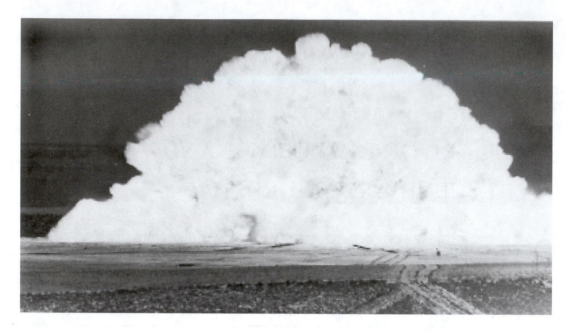

Figure 3-1 Detonation of 500 tons (454 metric tons) of TNT.

Modifying Factors

A number of factors can modify the effects of explosive blasts. Obviously, distance is the most important factor. The greater the distance from the detonation, the lower the peak overpressure. Sturdy barriers between the detonation and the target will afford some protection. Conversely, a detonation in a closed room or space will greatly amplify the effects of the blast.

TABLE 3-1

RELATIVE EXPLOSIVE POWER AND DETONATION VELOCITY
OF COMMONLY USED EXPLOSIVES

EXPLOSIVE	RELATIVE POWER	DETONATION VELOCITY, MILES/s (km/s)
TNT	1	3.2 – 4.3 (5.1 – 6.9)
Dynamite	0.9	2.5 – 4 (4 – 6)
C4	1.4	4.2 – 5 (6.8 – 8)
Ammonium nitrate/Fuel Oil	0.8	NA
PETN	1.3	4.9 (7.9)
Tetryl	1.2	4 (7)

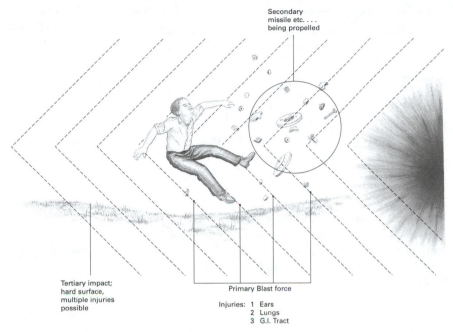

Secondary
missile etc. . . . .
being propelled

Tertiary impact;
hard surface,
multiple injuries
possible

Primary Blast force

Injuries: 1 Ears
          2 Lungs
          3 G.I. Tract

Figure 3-2 Multiple effects of blast on the human body.

Secondary Effects

The blast of an explosive is considered its primary effect. Flying debris, shrapnel and other projectiles are commonly associated with bombs. Theses high speed missiles can cause serious blunt or penetrating injury, and are referred to as secondary explosive effects (Figure 3-2). Flame or hot gases are present in all explosions and are another secondary effect. The victim's fall or flight as a result of the blast wave and resultant blunt trauma (when the body strikes the ground or a large object) are frequently referred to as tertiary explosive effects.

Body Position

Body position plays an important role in determining the extent of blast injury. Victims who are standing up or lying perpendicular to the blast will suffer the greatest injury, while victims lying directly toward or away from the blast suffer the least. Thus, if threatened by an imminent blast, immediately drop prone (on your stomach, face down) and face away from the expected detonation. This position minimizes blast effect and also creates a small cross-sectional profile, reducing associated shrapnel injury. For underwater blasts, floating on the surface is preferable to treading water, because body parts deeply immersed suffer the worst injuries. The patient's body position at the time of the detonation, as well as protective clothing or shelter will determine the extent of injuries from a bomb explosion.

The effects of a serious blast can cause injury to the lungs, abdomen, and ears (Figure 3-2). These injuries require special considerations regarding prehospital care.

Lungs

The history of exposure to the effects of a detonation should leave you suspicious of lung injury. Since it occurs more frequently and is more serious than abdominal and ear injury, any time you note such in a patient, suspect and rule out any lung involvement. The patient will frequently experience disturbances in the level of consciousness or small stroke-like symptoms. They may have dyspnea, and in extreme cases may display blood tinged sputum or cough up frank blood (hemoptysis).

If it becomes necessary to ventilate the blast injury patient, do so with caution. The mechanism of injury may damage the alveolar-capillary wall and open small blood vessels to the alveolar space. Positive pressure ventilation may push small air bubbles into the vascular system creating emboli. These emboli may quickly travel to the heart and brain where they can cause further injury or death. The pressure of ventilation may also induce pneumothorax by pushing air past blast induced defects in the lungs and into the pleural space.

Despite these risks, you should always provide artificial ventilation to blast injury patients with serious dyspnea. Use only the pressure needed to obtain moderate chest rise and respiratory volumes. High flow oxygen, as supplied with a reservoir, is also helpful because bubbles of oxygen in the blood stream are absorbed by the blood and less likely to cause injury than the nitrogen of room air.

Abdomen

Blast injury to the abdomen calls for no special attention in the early stages of care. The associated injuries, bowel hemorrhage and spillage of bowel contents will take some time before having an impact on the patient's overall condition. The only exception to this is when the blast is extremely powerful or the patient was very close to the detonation. In this case, look for evisceration of abdominal contents and provide rapid transportation and fluid resuscitation as needed.

Ears

The ears suffer greatly from the blast wave forces associated with ordnance explosion, artillery fire, and even repeated small arms fire at close range. The outer ear focuses the blast impact on the eardrum, causing irritation or rupture. If the blast is forceful, the delicate bones that transmit sound may fracture or dislocate. The patient may experience a temporary or permanent hearing loss. Care should support the patient and keep the ear canal uncontaminated. Often these injuries, even with as much as a third of the eardrum torn, will improve over time without much attention. The loss of hearing, however, may reduce the patient's ability to understand directions and recognize danger.

Blast injury can also result in extensive burn injury due either to the explosive charge ignition or ignition of fuels, clothing, or other munitions. Care of serious burn injury is discussed later in this chapter. Blast injury is also frequently associated with shrapnel and missile injury.

Assessment

The most immediately life-threatening result of blast injury is respiratory failure from lung injury. Lung tissue injury may result in bleeding, pulmonary edema or pneumothorax. Signs and symptoms include pain on respiration, dyspnea, hemoptysis, and respiratory failure. Auscultation may reveal crackles, decreased breath sounds diffusely, and if pneumothorax is present, decreased breath sounds over the affected lung.

Hollow organ (stomach, intestines, bladder) injury presents with abdominal pain, nausea, vomiting, hematemesis (bloody emesis) and shock. Entry wounds from shrapnel may be present. Tympanic membrane (ear drum) damage presents with ear pain, loss of hearing, tinnitus (ringing in the ears) and perhaps a trickle of blood in the external ear canal. Rarely, loss of balance or ataxia will occur.

Management

Treatment of primary blast injury is directed first at correcting imminent respiratory failure. Clear the airway with manual maneuvers, taking care to maintain cervical immobilization. Depending on the degree of airway compromise present, oral or nasopharyngeal airways, suction or orotracheal intubation may be indicated. If available, apply high flow oxygen by nonrebreather mask to all patients with dyspnea. Patients with severe respiratory distress or significant hypoxia require assisted ventilation with a bag-valve mask. Unfortunately, such blast-injury patients have a poor survival rate even with aggressive emergency care.

Simple pneumothorax is a significant risk of primary blast injury; tension pneumothorax is uncommon in this setting. Nonetheless, the signs of tension pneumothorax (including severe respiratory distress, hyperresonance to percussion and absent breath sounds on the affected side, tracheal deviation, distended neck veins, and hypotension) must be sought. If present, tension pneumothorax is immediately treated with needle decompression. Simple pneumothorax (absent or decreased breath sounds on the affected side without other serious signs) is treated with oxygen, nonocclusive dressings, reassurance and close monitoring for any changes.

Hollow organ injury requires no specific treatment beyond good supportive care and rapid transportation to definitive care. Administer high flow oxygen, initiate a large bore saline lock and keep the patient warm. If signs of uncompensated shock are present, administer 1000 ml normal saline bolus (20 ml/kg for children). Antibiotics and narcotic analgesics are withheld until directed by a physician. Do not give anything by mouth (npo) as the patient may require anesthesia and surgery for definitive management.

Tympanic membrane injury requires no specific therapy in the prehospital environment. The patient will require reassurance, however, since sudden hearing loss can create a sense of isolation and fright.

Triage

Triage of primary blast injury is dependent on the severity of injury and presenting problem. Patients with airway obstruction, respiratory distress and signs of uncompensated shock should be categorized as immediate. Hollow organ injury, with or without compensated shock are considered delayed. Most ambulatory patients including those with tympanic membrane damage and hearing loss will be categorized minimal. Respiratory failure, apnea and pulselessness are indications of poor survival and are therefore categorized as expectant.

Blast injury is rarely found in isolation. Instead, most patients will have associated injuries from falls, being struck by flying debris and shrapnel, and burns. Each of these possibilities must be considered during the focused and detailed assessment. These associated injuries are discussed later.

CRUSH INJURY

Crush injury refers to a pattern of trauma where a victim is subject to severe compressive forces. The usual cause is by being buried or crushed in a collapsed building. In the context of WMD, this may occur when buildings and other structures collapse and fall following some sort of explosion. The Oklahoma City bombing of the Federal Building is an example of this type of event. Other causes include cave-ins in mining and tunneling operations, collapse of trenches at construction sites, and building collapse from earthquakes and other natural disasters.

Mechanism

A bomb or other explosive device detonated in or near a building may cause sufficient damage to weaken or destroy the structural integrity of the structure. The building collapses, sending tons of debris raining down on any victims unlucky enough to be inside or nearby. The debris can be small rubble, larger chunks of concrete, or whole pieces of building. The net result is that the victim is trapped and crushed by tons of material and subject to severe compressive forces by the sheer weight of the debris.

Depending on the location and position of the victim, one or more extremities and the trunk may be crushed. The extent of the injury, as well as the specific body parts crushed, will largely determine the severity of injury and chance of survival.

Other Injury

Victims of crush injury from building collapse will frequently have other injuries. Falling debris will cause direct injury, both blunt and penetrating. Dust and smoke can cause respiratory and eye injuries. Entrapment for any length of time can lead to dehydration and hypothermia. All these possibilities must be considered when providing emergency care to victims of crush injury.

Pathophysiology

Crush syndrome can occur when body parts are entrapped for periods of four hours or longer. Shorter periods may certainly result in direct damage to the body part but usually do not cause the broad, systemic findings of crush syndrome. The crushed tissue undergoes necrosis and cellular changes with resultant release of metabolic by-products. Chief among these by-products is myoglobin (a muscle protein). Phosphate and potassium (from cellular death) and uric acid (from protein breakdown) are also released. These by-products accumulate in the crushed body part, but because of the entrapment, do not immediately reach the systemic circulation. However, once the victim is extricated and the pressure is released, the accumulated by-products and toxins flood into the rest of the circulation and cause serious problems.

High levels of myoglobin can accumulate in the filtering tubules of the kidney, leading to renal failure. Renal failure is a leading cause of delayed death in crush syndrome. More immediate problems include hypovolemia and shock from the influx of sodium, chloride and water from the damaged tissue. Hyperkalemia (increased blood potassium) can lead to cardiac dysrhythmias and sudden death. Hyperphosphatemia can lead to abnormal calcifications in the vasculature and nervous system and compound the problem.

Signs and Symptoms

Crush syndrome should be suspected in any victim entrapped (fallen building, cave-in, crashed automobile, etc.) for greater than four hours. The larger the body part or parts compressed and the longer the period of entrapment, the greater the risk of crush syndrome. Initially, the trapped patient will complain only of symptoms of the entrapment; pain, lack of motor function, tingling, or loss of sensation of the affected limb. With the body parts still trapped and the metabolic by-products still sequestered, the patient will not likely experience the full effects of crush syndrome.

Once extricated, however, the toxins are released and the patient may rapidly develop shock and die. If the patient survives the initial insult, there is still great risk of developing renal failure with serious morbidity or death.

Prehospital Management

The key to successful prehospital management of crush syndrome is anticipation of the problem and prevention of the effects. Since by definition all crush syndrome patients involve prolonged entrapment, most cases can be identified and treated before extrication is complete. The focus of prehospital care is on adequate fluid resuscitation and possibly, systemic alkalinization.

The prehospital approach to crush syndrome is similar to other forms of injury. Scene safety is paramount. Many victims will be buried in rubble or other large debris, and access may be difficult. Trained personnel and special equipment for urban search and rescue and confined space extrication may be needed. In any case, never place yourself or other rescuers in danger when attempting a rescue.

Once the scene is safe and the patient is reached, conduct an initial assessment. Remove debris from around the head, neck and thorax to minimize airway obstruction and restriction to ventilation. Control any obvious bleeding that can be reached. Perform a focused and detailed assessment, keeping in mind that portions of the patient's body will be inaccessible as a result of the entrapment. The dark, dusty and cramped conditions of many confined space rescues may force you to improvise.

Once you have assured the patient's ABCs, turn your attention to obtaining IV access. Intravenous fluids and selected medications are important in preventing and treating crush syndrome. Initiate two large bore IVs if possible. Because of the entrapment, it may be necessary to consider alternate IV sites such as the external jugular vein or the veins of the lower extremity. Avoid any site distal to a crush injury.

Infuse 1,000-2000 ml (20-40ml/kg) of normal saline, even in patients not showing signs of shock. Patients in shock will need additional fluid. Then, infuse normal saline at a rate of 1,500ml/hr (30ml/kg/hr) for as long as the patient remains trapped. Continue this infusion rate until the patient reaches the hospital. Avoid lactated ringers or other solutions containing potassium. The extra potassium can worsen the hyperkalemia associated with crush syndrome.

As in all patients receiving large volumes of crystalloid, periodically query the patient for symptoms of shortness of breath and auscultate the lungs for evidence of pulmonary edema (e.g. crackles). Stop or reduce the fluid rate if pulmonary edema is suspected. In young, healthy adults and children this will rarely occur at the fluid rates described here.

Alkalinization of the blood and urine is a consideration for preventing and treating crush syndrome. In combination with fluid resuscitation, alkalinization can help prevent renal failure and correct hyperkalemia. Administer sodium bicarbonate 1mEq/kg initially, followed by 0.25mEq/kg/hr thereafter. It is preferable to add the bicarbonate to the bag of normal saline rather than administering it as a bolus or IV push.

Cardiac (ECG) monitoring is important for all crush syndrome patients. Dysrhythmias are possible at anytime, but are most likely to occur immediately following the release of pressure with extrication. Sudden cardiac arrest should be treated in the usual fashion with defibrillation and cardiac drugs as appropriate. Calcium chloride 250-500mg (5-7 mg/kg) IV push may be used to counteract suspected hyperkalemia. An additional 1mEq/kg sodium bicarbonate should also be considered for the same reason. Be sure to flush the line between infusions because calcium chloride and sodium bicarbonate together will precipitate in the line.

Once the patient is freed from the entrapment, be prepared to treat rapidly progressing shock or sudden death. Continue the normal saline infusions at 30ml/kg/hr and provide additional boluses as needed. Rapid transport to an appropriate hospital (usually a trauma center) is indicated in most cases of suspected crush syndrome. If not already done, alert the receiving hospital so they can assemble the necessary personnel and equipment to manage the patient.

Prehospital care of the crushed limb or body parts requires no special technique. Cover open wounds on fractures, keeping in mind that progressive swelling will necessitate the adjustment of straps and splints. Handle all crushed limbs gently as the ischemic tissue is prone to injury. Elevation of severely crushed extremities is not indicated in the prehospital setting.

To harm a patient, a projectile must exchange its energy with the human tissue it contacts. To better understand the process of this exchange and the resultant bodily injury, we investigate the principles of kinetic energy and aspects of projectile travel that effect the rate of energy exchange. This energy exchange results in injury and is dependent upon both the nature of the projectile and the tissue it strikes. By examining projectile kinetic energy, the physical characteristics of energy exchange, the damage pathway, and the relative devastation projectile passage has on various body tissues and structures, we can better care for shrapnel wounds.

When a projectile strikes a target it exchanges its energy of motion, kinetic energy, with the object struck. This kinetic energy is the energy any object has when it is moving. It is related to two aspects of the object, its mass and its velocity. An object's mass (weight is the object's mass as pulled by gravity) has a direct and linear, relationship to its kinetic energy; the greater the mass, the greater the energy. If you double the mass of a bullet it has twice the kinetic energy if the speed remains the same. The speed (or velocity) of a projectile demonstrates a squared relationship to its energy. As the speed doubles, the energy increases fourfold. As the speed triples, the energy increases ninefold, and so on. The formula that describes this relationship is as follows:

$$\text{Kinetic Energy} = \frac{\text{Mass} \times \text{Velocity}^2}{2}$$

This relationship between mass and velocity explains why a very small and relatively light bullet traveling very fast, has the potential to do great damage. It also illustrates why faster, and to a lesser degree, heavier bullets have the ability to do greater damage. The same is true for shrapnel fragments. Most shrapnel is relatively small and with minimal mass. Since the fragment is irregularly shaped and expelled in all directions from the bomb, its velocity tends to be fairly low. Thus, most individual fragment wounds are not lethal unless a vital organ or large blood vessel is struck. Bombs compensate for this relatively low lethality by showering victims with hundreds of fragments, with deadly effects.

Energy Exchange

Objects traveling relatively slowly and without much kinetic energy will effect only the tissue they contact. This is true of most shrapnel fragments. Damage occurs as the projectile strikes tissue, contuses and tears it, and pushes it out of its way. The direct injury pathway is limited to the fragment profile as it moves through the body, or the profiles of resulting fragments as the piece breaks apart even further.

Tissue Damage

The extent of damage caused by a passing projectile is primarily dependent on the particular tissue it encounters. The density of an organ effects how efficiently the energy of projectile passage is transmitted to surrounding tissues. The connective strength and elasticity, called resiliency, also determine how much tissue damage occurs with the transfer of kinetic energy. Air is compressible and will absorb the pressure wave energy while fluids, which are not compressible, will transmit energy efficiently away from the point of impact. Structures and tissues within the body behaving differently during projectile passage include connective tissue, solid organs, hollow organs, lungs, and bone.

Connective Tissue

Muscle, the skin, and other connective tissues are dense, elastic, and held together very well. When struck by shrapnel these tissue characteristics absorb energy while limiting tissue damage. The wound track closes due to tissue resiliency and injury is frequently limited to the direct shrapnel pathway.

Solid Organs

Solid organs such as the liver, spleen, kidneys, and pancreas have the density but not the resiliency of muscle and other connective tissues. When subjected to shrapnel impact forces, the tissue compresses and stretches, resulting in greater damage. Hemorrhage associated with solid organ damage can be severe.

Hollow Organs

Hollow organs such as the bowel, stomach, urinary bladder, and heart are muscular containers holding fluid. When punctured by shrapnel, these organs can leak. In the case of the heart or great blood vessels, this can cause rapid and fatal blood loss. In the case of the gastrointestinal tract, the perforation will allow bowel contents to leak, setting the stage for a delayed but severe peritonitis and septic shock.

Lungs

The lungs consist of millions of small elastic air-filled sacs. The fragment may open the chest wall or disrupt larger airways, permitting air to escape into the thorax (pneumothorax). The injury may form a valve-like opening, accumulating pressure within the chest (tension pneumothorax).

Bone

In contrast to lung tissue, bone is the densest, most rigid, and non-elastic body tissue of all. When impacted by a projectile, bone resists displacement until it fractures, often into numerous pieces. These bone fragments then may absorb the energy of impact and become projectiles themselves, extending the area of tissue damage.

The particular organ involved in a penetrating injury also has profound effects on the patient's potential for survival. Some organs, like the heart, are immediately necessary, and serious injury may not be survivable. Penetrating injury of the urinary bladder, on the other hand, may allow survival for many hours without surgical intervention. When evaluating the seriousness of a wound, anticipate the organs injured and their impact on the patient's condition and survivability.

Assessment

When evaluating a victim of an explosive detonation, consider the likelihood of shrapnel injury. Victims close to the detonation will likely have primary blast and burn wounds as their most serious problem, while those further away will more likely be suffering primarily shrapnel wounds. Focus your initial assessment in the usual fashion. Airway obstruction from facial damage or airway injury must be rapidly identified and treated. Visual evidence includes obvious face or head injury. Stridor and gurgling respirations are strong aural clues to potential obstruction. Evaluate all shrapnel victims for potential tension pneumothorax, even if no chest wounds are seen. The shrapnel fragment may be small and create an unnoticeable entry wound. Because of the possibility of shrapnel wounds anywhere on the body, a thorough head-to-toe examination is required once the initial assessment is complete.

Management

Treatment of shrapnel wounds should be guided by the suspected injuries from the projectile. Secure the airway in any patient with imminent airway compromise. Provide high flow supplemental oxygen at 12-15 lpm and initiate at least one large bore IV. Respiratory failure is treated with overdrive (assisted) ventilations. Be prepared to immediately decompress tension pneumothorax if one is suspected. Control all significant external bleeding with direct pressure.

Apply dry sterile dressings to all wounds. Hypovolemic shock is treated with fluid administration, usually normal saline. If shock is present and all bleeding is felt to be controlled, administer 1,000 ml (20 ml/kg) fluid boluses up to 3,000 ml (60 ml/kg). In cases where shock is present and the suspected cause is uncontrolled intra-abdominal or intrathoracic bleeding, administer 1,000 ml (20 ml/kg) only. While controversial, many experts feel that exceeding these values can be counterproductive. Victims of penetrating injury and uncontrolled intra-abdominal or intrathoracic bleeding require prompt transport to a facility with general and thoracic surgery capabilities.

Triage

No special rules apply to the triage of patients with shrapnel wounds. Potentially correctable airway obstruction, respiratory distress, and uncontrolled hemorrhage would ordinarily be considered immediate. Less serious head, neck, trunk and some extremity wounds (those with lots of damage or functional loss) might be categorized as delayed, as they may need surgery, although not urgently. Those with minor wounds are considered minimal. Apnea, pulselessness and injuries incompatible with life are considered expectant.

INCENDIARY AND BURN INJURIES

Incendiary devices and munitions include napalm, thermite and white phosphorous. While these weapons are neither new or unconventional, they do produce injury patterns sufficiently different from conventional bombs to warrant separate discussion (Figure 3-3).

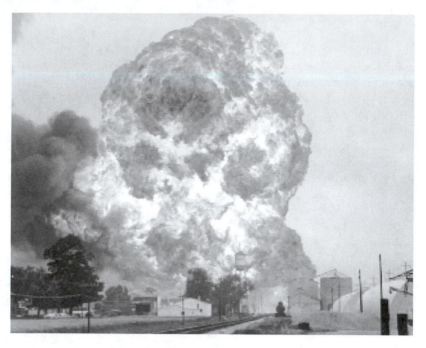

Figure 3-3 Flame and incendiary devices can produce a spectrum of injuries.

There are many types of incendiary devices. Table 3-2 lists four common types of materials used to produce the incendiary effect. Most incendiary devices are designed to be employed against equipment. Some, such as napalm, are designed to be used against personnel.

Incendiary devices are designed to burn at very high temperatures. This burning process is the primary mechanism of injury. Magnesium burns the hottest, and it is capable of rapidly melting through steel. Thermite burns at slightly lower temperatures. Any individuals in the vicinity of these munitions will likely suffer severe burns.

Napalm (and its close cousin, gasoline) burns at a lower temperature, but its employment against personnel will frequently result in many more burns than result from other devices. The simple "malotov cocktail" is an inexpensive gasoline incendiary device in use for over 75 years. White phosphorous deserves special mention because it can spontaneously combust in air.

Mechanism of Burns

Thermal burns are caused by contact with material hot enough to cause damage. It can also be caused by exposure to energy of sufficient strength. Hot gases, including steam, flames, electricity, laser beams and microwave energy are examples of burn causing agents. The common result of these agents is damage and destruction of the skin and other bodily structures.

TABLE 3-2

TYPES OF INCENDIARY MATERIALS

TYPE	BURNING TEMPERATURE °C
Napalm	1000
Thermite	2,000 - 3,000
Magnesium	3,000
White Phosphorous	800

Medical Effects

The medical effects of these burn-causing agents are no different than those found in traditional prehospital care. The primary organ system affected by burns is the skin (Figure 3-4). Initially, the skin reddens (erythema) and becomes painful (first degree burn). As damage progresses, the skin blisters and swells (second degree burn). Because only the outer layers of skin are destroyed in first and second degree burns, these are sometimes termed partial-thickness burns. Further damage destroys all skin layers and results in charred, painless areas (third degree burn) also termed full-thickness burns. Second and third degree burned skin swells and "leaks" large amounts of fluid, accounting for the need to provide intravenous fluids. Further burning will damage deeper structures such as muscle, blood vessels, bone, and vital organs.

Other organ systems affected by burns include the upper airway (respiratory tract), lungs and eyes. Airway burns may result in rapidly life-threatening swelling and obstruction. Signs of potential airway burns are listed in Table 3-3. Stridor is a particularly ominous sign and demands immediate attention. Lower respiratory tract (lung) burns are rare but can be caused by super-heated steam. Signs include dyspnea, cough, and crackles from pulmonary edema. Eye burns can result in vision loss. Pain, conjunctival erythema ("red eye"), tearing and blurry vision are likely signs.

Body Surface Area

A key principle in determining the extent of a burn is estimating the total body surface area (BSA) affected by second or third degree burns (first degree burns are not counted). Figure 3-5 illustrates the proportion of each body area. With practice, the EMS provider should be able to make burn estimates on a given patient in under one minute. Within reason, accuracy is important, since prehospital treatment and triage largely depend on good estimates of the total BSA burned.

Assessment

Prehospital management of incendiary or flame munitions injury is the same as for any burn. The first priority is to stop the burning process, if necessary. Immediately smother

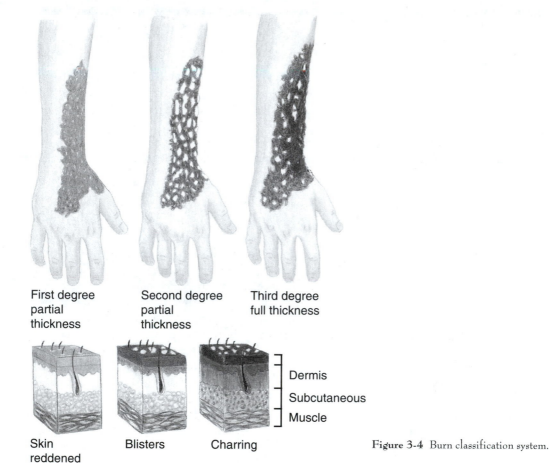

First degree
partial
thickness

Second degree
partial
thickness

Third degree
full thickness

Dermis

Subcutaneous

Muscle

Skin
reddened

Blisters

Charring

Figure 3-4 Burn classification system.

TABLE 3-3

SIGNS OF POTENTIAL AIRWAY BURNS

- Stridor
- Oropharyngeal Swelling
- Hoarseness
- Drooling
- Difficulty Swallowing
- Carbonaceous sputum
- Singed nasal or facial hair
- Dyspnea

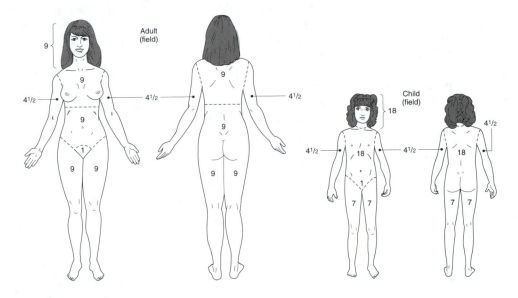

Figure 3-5 Rule of 9s to estimate body surface area.

flames by wrapping the patient in a blanket or by rolling on the ground. If available, copious water is very effective in stopping the burning process.

Once the burning process is stopped, the focus of the initial assessment is on airway patency and adequacy of respirations. Facial burns, singed facial hair, sooty, carbonaceous sputum or oropharyngeal swelling are all sign of possible airway burns. Tachypnea (respiratory rate >24 in an adult or > 60 in an infant) and stridor (high-pitched "whooping" sound heard on each inspiration) are particularly ominous.

Focused assessment includes and estimation of body surface area burned and the degree or depth of burns. In the detailed assessment, search for associated blast, missile or fragment wounds that may accompany incendiary detonations.

Management

The general prehospital management of burns applies to the WMD incident. Readers requiring a thorough review of general burn care are encouraged to consult any one of the many good emergency care texts available. A brief synopsis will be presented here.

The first step in burn care is to stop the burning process. Immediately smother any flames with a jacket, blanket or available material. Water is exceptionally useful as it simultaneously smothers flames and cools hot tissue. Rolling the patient on the ground is also effective.

Once the burning has stopped, perform an initial assessment. Concentrate on the airway, as this is the area most imminently threatened by burns. Skin burns themselves are not immediately fatal and can wait until other priorities are addressed. Patients exhibiting severe respiratory compromise will require assisted (overdrive) ventilations.

Intubation is indicated for patients exhibiting severe airway compromise including severe dyspnea, stridor and oropharyngeal swelling. If intubation is not feasible, manual airway maneuvers (jaw thrust, chin lift techniques, etc.) may buy sufficient time until the patient reaches additional care. On rare occasions, a surgical airway may be lifesaving in the face of severe upper airway swelling from burns. High flow (12-15 lpm) supplemental oxygen using a nonrebreather mask is indicated for any patient with dyspnea.

Remove the patient's clothing and gear for the focused and detailed assessments. Keep the patient warm, as burned skin is unable to properly maintain body temperature. Estimate the total BSA burned.

Cover all second and third degree burns with dry, sterile dressings. Do not apply ointments or creams unless directed by a physician. Initiate a large bore saline lock (two if signs of shock are present) and administer fluid as described below. Burns can be extremely painful and parenteral narcotic analgesia is indicated.

Fluid Resuscitation

Severe burns require fluid resuscitation. The choice of fluid (normal saline, lactated ringers, colloid solutions) is the subject of ongoing discussion and research. To date, the optimal fluid for burn resuscitation is not identified. Nonetheless, normal saline can be recommended because of its effectiveness, availability and cost. Lactated Ringers is an acceptable alternative and can be substituted one-for-one with normal saline.

All burn patients exhibiting signs of uncompensated shock should receive an immediate bolus of 1000 ml (20 ml/kg) of saline. Patients with a BSA > 20% (10% for children) will require additional fluid, even if signs of shock are absent. However, if transport times are short (≤ two hours), this can be safely deferred until the patient reaches more definitive care.

If transport times are long (>two hours), patients with a total BSA greater than 20% (10% for children) will require additional fluid to be administered by the EMS provider. For the first 4 hours of evacuation delay administer fluid according to the following formula:

0.5 ml normal saline x patient weight (kg) x total BSA burned.

This amount may be repeated if the delay extends for four to eight hours. For even longer delays, the amount of fluid administered (using the formula) is the same, but the timing interval increases. Thus, for a delay of eight to sixteen hours, the fluid dose may be repeated a third time and for sixteen to twenty-four hours, repeated a fourth time. In twenty-four hours, the patient should receive:

2 ml normal saline x patient weight (kg) x total BSA burned.

Ideally, the fluid should be administered as a drip. However, for the adult, it is acceptable to divide the fluid dose into 1000 ml boluses and administer them individually.

Serious burns are quite painful and morphine 2 mg IV/IM should be administered. This dose may be repeated as needed. Medication endpoints are relief of suffering (not elimination of all pain) or untoward side effects, including decreased level of consciousness, hypotension or respiratory depression.

Care for minor burns ($1° < 20\%$, $2°/3° < 5\%$) includes dry, sterile dressings and elevation of the affected part (e.g., hands or feet). Elevation can significantly reduce swelling and is indicated for all but the most trivial burns. Referral of the patient to the physician is required, but may be safely delayed for minor burns until the incident is under control.

White phosphorous (WP) burns deserve special note because WP combusts spontaneously in air. On occasion, a patient will be showered with WP fragments from a nearby explosion. This WP "shrapnel" can become imbedded in the skin and continue to burn. Treatment includes covering the WP with water. If possible, submerge the affected body part in lukewarm (not hot or cold) water. Alternatively, use saline-soaked bandages to cover the wounds. Keep the WP covered with water until the patient reaches definitive care.

Triage

Potential airway obstruction and dyspnea are critical markers of significant burn injury and warrant an immediate categorization. First and second degree burns greater than 20% body surface area of an adult ordinarily would be considered delayed. Less than 20% second/third degree burns would be minimal. Serious, whole body burns greater than 70% in a young adult (50% in an older or chronically ill individual) are likely lethal, and therefore such patients can be classified as expectant.

SUMMARY

Blast and burn injuries represent significant modern threats and all EMS providers must be proficient in treating these patients. Knowledge and understanding of the basic mechanisms of injury coupled with a recognition of key signs and symptoms is important to the successful field treatment of these patients.

FOR FURTHER READING

BELLAMY RF, et al (eds): Conventional Warfare: Ballistic, Blast and Burn Injuries, Department of the Army, Washington, D.C. 1991

BOWEN TE, et al: Emergency War Surgery, 2nd Ed, U.S. Government Printing Office, Washington, D.C. 1988

TRUNKEY DD, et al: Management of Battle Casualties, in Feliziano DV, et al (eds): Trauma, 3rd Ed. Appleton & Lang, Stamford, CT 1996

MONAFO WM: Initial Management of Burns. N Engl J Med 1996; 335(21): 1581-1586

MEYER EUGENE: Chemistry of Hazardous Materials, 3rd Ed. Prentice-Hall, Upper Saddle River, NJ 1998

4

CARE OF CHEMICAL AGENT INJURIES

INTRODUCTION

Chemical weapons can be among the most terrifying of all weapons of mass destruction. Yet with proper training and equipment, it is possible to operate in a chemically contaminated environment and perform basic patient care. This chapter will review the medical effects of chemical weapons, emergency field treatment, and expedient decontamination of patients. Additionally, the use of self-protective masks, garments and other equipment will be reviewed.

History

Although thought of as a modern invention, chemical weapons date back to ancient times. In the Peloponnesian War in 423 BC, smoke was used against an Athens, Greece fort. In this century, poison gas was used by both Germany and Britain in WWI. Although chemical weapons were not decisive in the war, the psychological shock as well as the blinding and choking injuries were devastating.

Following WWI, most nations were so horrified by the use of poison gas that its use was outlawed by international treaty. To date, this treaty has been successful in preventing large-scale chemical weapons use. In 1997, a new treaty banned not only the use but also the manufacture of chemical weapons.

Current Threat

Revelations of recent chemical weapons manufacture by Iraq and limited use by the former Soviet Union and Cambodia renewed concern among prehospital medical providers that they might face chemical agent injuries. The specter of a terrorist attack against civilians using chemical weapons was underscored by the sarin nerve gas attack on a Tokyo subway in 1996. Terrorist groups can acquire or manufacture chemical weapons with relative ease, and it is now imperative that all EMS providers be familiar with chemical patient management.

To care properly for patients of chemical agents, it is important to understand the nature and properties of the chemicals. With a basic knowledge of chemical agents, the EMS provider can anticipate the type and severity of injuries expected. Furthermore, by understanding how chemical agents are deployed and used, the EMS provider can better protect against personal injury when working in a contaminated environment or on exposed patients. Table 1-4 (chapter 1, Medical Aspects of WMD) outlines some important characteristics of chemical agents.

Solids, Liquids, and Gases

Most chemical weapons are stored in munitions (shells, rockets, and bombs) as a liquid. When the munition explodes, the liquid turns into an aerosol, or tiny droplets of liquid suspended in the air. A terrorist might simply release the agent into a closed building or disperse it in the open air. A crude munition could be built by attaching a small bomb to a chemical agent canister, allowing the agent to be dispersed when the bomb explodes. A few riot control agents are stored as solids, but like liquid agents become aerosols after deployment. Thus "tear gas" is not a gas at all, but aerosolized solid agent. Likewise, "mustard gas" is a liquid suspended in the air. These properties of chemical agents will become important when chemical defense and decontamination are discussed later in the chapter.

Volatility and Persistence

Some agents, such as hydrogen cyanide, chlorine, and phosgene, may be gases during warm weather. Other agents, such as nerve and mustard, are liquids at these temperatures but will evaporate like a puddle of water. This tendency to evaporate is called volatility. A volatile liquid evaporates easily, rapidly forming a dangerous, breathable vapor. The opposite of volatility is persistence. Agents that tend not to evaporate quickly remain as concentrated, dangerous puddles and droplets on surfaces. Because of this, they may remain hazardous to touch for days or weeks after deployment. In general, the warmer the temperatures, the greater the evaporation (and danger from breathing vapors), and the colder the temperature, the greater the persistence (and danger from direct contact) of the agent.

Portal of Entry

Chemical agents in the form of aerosolized liquids or solids, vapor, or gas can enter the body through the respiratory tract (lungs), eyes, or skin. The lungs are by far the most important route for these agents. While local damage to the lungs, eyes, and skin is also possible, the large absorptive area of the lungs allows large quantities of aerosols, vapors, and gases to enter the body. Thus, severe systemic affects are possible by this route.

Liquid agents tend to be absorbed primarily through the skin and eyes. Both severe local effect (chemical burns) and serious systemic effects are possible. Although infrequently encountered, accidental ingestion of chemical agents (e.g., eating contaminated food) can also lead to serious local and systemic effects. The specific effects of various chemical agents will be discussed in the following section.

Types of Chemical Agents

There are five major types of chemical agents which will be discussed: 1) nerve agents, 2) vesicants, 3) cyanide, 4) pulmonary agents, and 5) riot control agents. For each class of agent, the toxicity, signs and symptoms, emergency care, triage, and decision making will be discussed.

NERVE AGENTS

Overview

Nerve agents are among the deadliest compounds known to man (Table 4-1). Because of this lethality, nerve agents represent the biggest threat to troops and noncombatants alike on the chemical battlefield. Because of their potency and relatively easy manufacture, they make similarly deadly weapons in the hands of terrorists. All EMS providers need to be familiar with these agents and their effects.

Nerve agents were invented by the Germans in WWII, though they were never used. The U.S. currently has the agents GB and VX in its inventory, but is committed to destroying this stockpile over the next decade or so. The technology to manufacture, store and deploy nerve agents is not terribly complex, and many rogue nations are believed to have this technical capability.

Nerve agents are liquid under most weather conditions. When dispersed, the more volatile ones represent both a vapor and liquid hazard. The least volatile agents are VX and GF. Both are persistent agents and represent mostly a liquid hazard.

Toxicity

Nerve agents exert their toxic effects by inhibiting or blocking the action of acetylcholinesterase, a critical enzyme. Acetylcholinesterase (AChE) is found in the plasma, red blood cells and nervous tissue. Although nerve agents will affect the enzyme in all three areas, it is the neurological effects which are most important and will be the focus of this discussion.

TABLE 4-1

LETHAL DOSES* OF VARIOUS NERVE AGENTS

AGENT	SKIN DOSE, MG	VAPOR DOSE, MG-MIN/M3
GA (tabun)	1000	400
GB (sarin)	1700	100
GD (soman)	50	70
GF	30	unknown
VX	10	50

*50% fatality rate, other 50% severely incapacitated

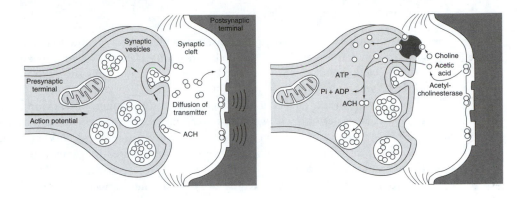

Figure 4-1 Synapse showing acetylcholine flowing across the synapse to excite the end organ (muscle, gland or nerve), and AChE rapidly metabolizing the acetylcholine into inactive substances.

Acetylcholine, a neurotransmitter, functions primarily in the smooth and skeletal muscles, the central nervous system, and glands. It's action is to excite or turn "on" the muscle, gland or nerve across the synapse, or connection (Figure 4-1). To excite the end organ (e.g., skeletal muscle), the nerve ending releases acetylcholine into the synapse and the muscle contracts. The muscle will continue to contract as long as acetylcholine is present, so to release the muscle contraction, a special enzyme called acetylcholinesterase (AChE) rapidly metabolizes the acetylcholine into inactive substances. This turns the muscle "off." Normally, the "on-off" process is very rapid and efficient and allows for effective control over muscles.

A nerve agent works by blocking or inhibiting the action of AChE. This allows acetylcholine to rapidly build up in the synapse, causing it to remain in the "on" state. The net effect on muscles at first is uncontrolled and uncoordinated contraction of the muscle fibers. This is seen as fasciculations. Shortly afterward, the muscles fatigue and cease to work. Death usually results from respiratory muscle failure.

Nerve agents are extremely potent blockers of AChE. Only small amounts (Table 4-1) are needed to effectively block all the AChE in the body and produce serious consequences. Several medications exist which can break the bond between the nerve agent and AChE, thus regenerating the AChE. Unfortunately, over a period of time (minutes to hours) the nerve agent becomes permanently attached to the AChE, preventing any regeneration. This "aging" process will markedly reduce the effectiveness of antidotal therapy, making early use of proper antidotes critical in the treatment of nerve agent poisoning.

Several compounds exist which are related to nerve agents but are much less deadly. The most common of these are the organophosphate and carbamate insecticides, and medications. These compounds will cause symptoms similar to those of nerve agents, and in large doses can resemble acute nerve agent poisoning. Organophosphates and carbamates do not, however, permanently bind to AChE. The principles of care outlined in this section for nerve agents will also apply to organophosphate and carbamate poisonings.

Assessment

The signs and symptoms of nerve agent poisoning will depend on the dose and route of exposure. In general, larger doses and direct breathing of nerve agent vapor results in quicker onset and greater severity of effects. Table 4-2 summarizes the signs and symptoms of nerve agent exposure.

The most important effects of nerve agents are on the lungs, airways, and the nervous system. Large doses of nerve agent will wreak havoc with the brain's ability to function and result in rapid loss of consciousness, convulsions (seizures) and apnea. Lower doses can result in difficulty concentrating, insomnia, impaired judgement, and depression. Hallucinations and confusion do not occur.

The pulmonary system is affected by two separate mechanisms that together often contribute to death. First is respiratory failure from paralysis of the respiratory muscles (diaphragm, abdominal, and thoracic muscles). The result is apnea. The second mechanism is copious airway secretions leading to obstructed larger airways and bronchoconstriction leading to obstruction of the smaller airways. The patient may be drooling or pooling secretions in the oropharynx. Wheezing may be prominent if air exchange is still good, or diminished if respiratory failure ensues.

Other clinical effects of nerve agents are less important but can give important clues to the cause of the poisoning. Perhaps most characteristic are pinpoint pupils or miosis. This finding, in combination with the right prehospital setting and other suspicious symptoms, can lead the EMS provider to suspect nerve agent exposure. Other less characteristic signs and symptoms include runny nose (rhinorrhea), copious salivation, tearing of the eyes, blurry vision, nausea and vomiting, diarrhea, sweating, and loss of bladder control. The nemonic SLUDGE helps identify some of these findings. It stands for Salivation, Lacrimation, Urination, Defecation, and Gastric Emptying. Initially, vital signs may reflect tachypnea (rapid breathing), tachycardia, or bradycardia (either fast or slow pulse) and normal blood pressure. Later, as effects worsen to life-threatening levels, the patient will usually have apnea, tachycardia and hypotension (low blood pressure).

TABLE 4-2

SIGNS AND SYMPTOMS OF NERVE AGENT EXPOSURE

VAPOR	small exposure	miosis, rhinorrhea, mild dyspnea
	large exposure	sudden unconsciousness, convulsions, apnea, copious secretions, miosis
LIQUID	small exposure	localized sweating, nausea, vomiting, fatigue
	large exposure	sudden unconsciousness, convulsions, apnea, paralysis, copious secretions

---

Identification of an Attack

The early signs of a nerve agent attack are the same clinical signs and symptoms mentioned in the preceding paragraphs. All EMS personnel should be alert for these signs. Before the nerve agent has reached incapacitating levels, most victims will experience blurry vision, runny nose, feelings of tightness in the chest, and mild weakness or fatigue. Additionally, animals will also be affected by the agent. Insects, birds and small animals will all show varying degrees of effects. If you should notice these signs in patients, bystanders or wildlife, sound the alarm. These early effects serve as a warning signal. All rescue team members must don their chemical protective gear first, and then consider injecting themselves with a single Mark I antidote if exposure is likely.

EMERGENCY CARE

The first action when encountering a suspected nerve agent patient is to protect yourself and your team from exposure. The patient should also be protected from further exposure through decontamination (see chapter 7, Personal Protection and Patient Decontamination). The usual measures of basic and advanced life support apply for chemical patients. This section will highlight the key elements of treating and resuscitating victims of chemical agents (Table 4-3).

TABLE 4-3

KEY MEASURES IN RESUSCITATING NERVE AGENT PATIENTS

- Secure airway and provide positive pressure ventilation
- Administer atropine and pralidoxime
- Administer diazepam
- Repeat atropine and pralidoxime as needed

Initial resuscitation

Initial resuscitation should be directed at obtaining an airway and providing adequate ventilation. If possible, intubate the patient orally. Portable suction may be needed to clear the oropharynx of pooled secretions. If unable to intubate, an oral or nasopharyngeal airway in combination with the jaw-thrust or head-tilt, chin-lift manual method will work. Provide positive pressure ventilation at a rate of 20 breaths/min for an adult patient. Position the patient in the recovery position (preferred) or supine.

Antidotes

The next key step in the resuscitation is the administration of an antidote. Currently, two drugs are available to counter the effects of nerve agents: atropine and pralidoxime

(2-pam-chloride or Protopam). Atropine, an anticholinergic, works by blocking the effect of excess acetylcholine at peripheral nervous synapses. This reduces the effects of the nerve agent. In particular, secretions will be reduced and ventilation will be easier. For early symptoms, self-administration of atropine is indicated. Atropine is administered in 2 mg increments up to a total of 12 mg. The preferred route is intravenously. Intramuscular, or if necessary, endotracheal administration is acceptable. The pediatric dose is 0.02 mg/kg increments (0.1 mg minimum dose to avoid paradoxical bradycardia) up to a total of 0.12 mg/kg.

Pralidoxime works by breaking the bond between the nerve agent and AChE, thus regenerating the AChE. Pralidoxime is only able to work if the bond has not "aged" and become permanent. Different nerve agents "age" at different rates (minutes to hours) with GD (soman) bonding permanently within two minutes. Pralidoxime does not work as rapidly as atropine, so it is usually administered simultaneously with each dose of atropine. The adult dosage of pralidoxime is 600 mg IV/IM for mild symptoms and 1800 mg IV/IM for severe symptoms. The pediatric dosage is 25 mg/kg up to 600 mg for mild symptoms and 50 mg/kg for severe symptoms, also by the IV/IM route. A rational

TABLE 4-4

GUIDELINES FOR INITIAL ANTIDOTE DOSING IN NERVE AGENT EXPOSURES FOR ADULTS
(SEE TEXT FOR PEDIATRIC DOSES.)

SYMPTOMS	WHO ADMINISTERS	DRUG	ROUTE
MILD Miosis, blurry vision, mild dyspnea, runny nose	self, or EMS provider	atropine 2 mg plus pralidoxime 600 mg (one Mark I). Repeat in ten minutes if not improved (two Mark Is total)	autoinjector
SEVERE Above, plus severe dyspnea, generalized fasciculations, convulsions, unconscious	EMS Provider	atropine 6 mg plus pralidoxime 1800 mg (three Mark Is), plus Diazepam 10 mg	autoinjector, IV,IM autoinjector IV,IM
Continued resuscitation	EMS provider	above, plus atropine 2 mg every five minutes up to 20 mg total Diazepam 5 mg every five minutes up to 20 mg total	IV, IM, ET or autoinjector IV, IM, ET or autoinjector

TABLE 4-5

GUIDELINES FOR CONTINUED DOSING IN CHEMICAL AGENT
EXPOSURES WITH SEVERE SYMPTOMS
(SEVERE DYSPNEA, CONVULSIONS, UNCONSCIOUSNESS)
ADULT DOSAGES SEE TEXT FOR PEDIATRIC DOSAGES.

DRUG	DOSE	INTERVAL	PREFERRED ROUTE	ENDPOINT
Atropine	2 mg	5 min	IV (or IM, ET)	Drying of secretions or 20 mg
Pralidoxime	1 gm	60 min	IV (or IM) over 20 min	Spontaneous respirations
Diazepam	10 mg	2-3 hrs	IV (or IM/ET)	Seizure control

approach to antidote dosing is given in Table 4-4. These guidelines were modified from military recommendations to include the capabilities of advanced level providers.

It is important to monitor the patient for a response when using atropine and pralidoxime in a nerve agent poisoning. Gauge the need for additional dosing by the patient's signs and symptoms. A drying of the secretions indicates adequate atropinization, while continued copious secretions indicate a need for more atropine. In a similar fashion, the appropriate endpoint for pralidoxime administration is the return of spontaneous respirations. Table 4-5 outlines these endpoints and provides guidelines for the continued dosing of drugs if the patient remains in the field or undergoes prolonged transport.

A third medication, diazepam (Valium), is useful in the resuscitation of chemical patients. Diazepam does not directly counteract the nerve agent, but instead treats or reduces the likelihood of convulsions or seizures. Other benzodiazepines such as lorazepam (Ativan) are equally effective and may be substituted at the appropriate doses. Unlike atropine and pralidoxime, diazepam and other benzodiazepines are never self-administered. A patient needing diazepam would be incapacitated and thus unable to self-administer it. Diazepam is administered as an initial 10 mg slow IV push or IM injection. It may also be administered down the endotracheal tube. The pediatric dose is 0.2 mg/kg up to 10 mg IV/IM/ET.

Autoinjectors

Atropine, pralidoxime and diazepam are all available in autoinjector form (Figure 4-2) for easy administration. Standard military doctrine calls for each soldier to carry three autoinjectors of atropine and pralidoxime for self-injection. The military medic can also inject the casualty using the casualty's autoinjectors if necessary. One autoinjector of valium is also carried, but this is for use by the soldier's buddy or by a medic, since any casualty needing diazepam would not be able to self-administer it.

The EMS provider can certainly use the autoinjectors to treat patients if available. Autoinjectors are a rapid method of administering antidotes. However, the intramuscular route (autoinjectors use this route) is not ideal. If time and circumstances permit, an IV should be started and atropine, pralidoxime and diazepam administered IV. Atropine and diazepam can also be administered through the endotracheal tube, if necessary. EMS providers and other rescuers should also consider carrying three Mark I autoinfectors on

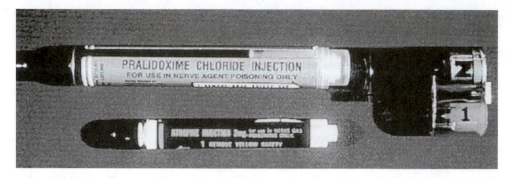

Figure 4-2 Military Mark I autoinjector kit.

their person whenever operating in a possible nerve-agent contaminated area. Self-treatment should be initiated for any symptoms compatible with nerve agent poisoning.

Additional Concerns

Injuries or wounds from conventional weapons should be treated in the usual fashion with attention to decontaminating and covering wounds to prevent further absorption of nerve agent. Keep the patient warm and evacuate as soon as possible.

Individuals with small exposures may develop only mild effects, such as shortness of breath, blurry vision, runny nose, tearing and fatigue. Aggressive treatment with antidotes is warranted, and these patients will likely demonstrate some improvement. However, since the antidotes themselves (particularly atropine) cause uncomfortable and sometimes incapacitating effects, these patients will also need to be transported.

There is concern voiced by a few experts about administering the first dose of atropine by the IM route, rather than the IV route. Because the heart is relatively hypoxic and sensitized by the nerve agent, there is a theoretical risk of causing dysrhythmias in the heart. However, data to support this assertion is scant, and most authorities agree that intravenous atropine is safe and effective.

If the nerve agent exposure is not too large and the patient receives prompt treatment, the chances of survival are good. Early antidote administration is vital, as is continued support of ventilation. If at all possible, begin antidotal therapy using autoinjectors even before decontamination is complete. The autoinjector can be used even if the patient is wearing a full protective ensemble (Figure 4-3). The sharp steel needle will easily penetrate several layers of clothing. If resuscitation is prompt, modest improvement can be expected in a few hours. The patient will begin spontaneously breathing and will require less atropine to control secretions. The patient's level of consciousness will improve, although he will remain intermittently obtunded and very weak. Care at this point includes administration of supplemental oxygen, keeping the patient warm, and prompt transportation.

Triage and Decision Making

The principles of triage for nerve agent patients are the same as those for conventional patients. Nerve agent patients with severe difficulty breathing, apnea, unconsciousness,

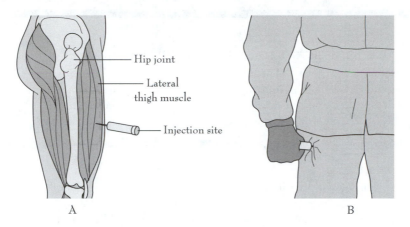

A   B

Figure 4-3 Self-injecting nerve agent antidote using Mark I autoinjector.

or convulsions would be considered immediate. If possible, securing of the airway and breathing followed by antidotal therapy should begin immediately. If, however, the patient has no pulse or blood pressure, he would not be expected to survive even with aggressive therapy. This patient would be considered expectant.

A patient with severe symptoms who is conscious and breathing has an excellent chance of survival. The triage category of immediate is appropriate with initial therapy consisting of the administration of three Mark I kits plus one valium autoinjector. Such therapy is effective in this situation and requires only one or two minutes to accomplish. The patient should, however, be watched for worsening of his condition.

Ambulatory or walking patients are considered minimal. However, they should be instructed to self-administer one Mark I autoinjector (Figure 4-3) and then be observed for any changes. If symptoms do not worsen, or better yet, improve in several hours, many of these patients can assist in the recovery operation, although their effectiveness will be diminished. In a mass casualty incident, these individuals could be expected to take a bus or truck, or perhaps walk to the hospital.

VESICANTS

Overview

Vesicants are a group of chemical agents that cause damage to exposed skin, lungs, eyes, and can also cause generalized illness if a significant amount is absorbed. Vesicants date back to WWI when sulfur mustard was first used. The current threat includes sulfur and nitrogen mustards, lewisite and phosgene oxide (Table 4-6). All these agents will cause localized blistering, burning and tissue damage on contact. The eyes, skin, and lungs are the most commonly affected organs. The key difference between the mustard agents and the others is in the onset of effects. Lewisite and phosgene oxime produce immediate pain and redness on contact. Mustard, however, causes little initial discomfort but will

TABLE 4-6

CURRENT VESICANT AGENTS AND ONSET OF SYMPTOMS

HD	sulfur mustard	delayed
HN	Nitrogen mustard	delayed
L	Lewisite	immediate
CX	Phosgene oxime	immediate

cause severe damage within a few hours. Vesicants can cause systemic or generalized illness if significant amounts are absorbed.

All vesicants except phosgene oxime are thick, oily liquids. They have low volatility and hence tend to be persistent. In warm temperatures, vesicants pose a significant vapor hazard. Mustard has an odor of onions, garlic, or mustard while phosgene oxime smells of newly mown grass or hay. However, the sense of smell is unreliable and should never be relied upon for chemical agent detection.

Toxicity

Vesicant agents cause damage on contact. The agent causes local damage at the cellular level, leading to tissue destruction. Blisters commonly form, hence the old term "blister agent." Mucous membranes, particularly the eyes and respiratory tract, are very sensitive to vesicants. The net result is a chemical burn of the affected area.

Vesicants can also be absorbed into the body and bloodstream and cause systemic damage. Mustard in particular will damage the blood-forming organs (bone marrow) and can cause life-threatening illness days or weeks after the initial skin injury. However, the body fluids of vesicant patients do not contain hazardous levels of the agent and no special precautions are needed beyond standard universal precautions.

Assessment

Vesicant agents cause burning, redness (erythema), blisterings and necrosis of exposed skin. Eye contact results in stinging, tearing and development of eyesight-threatening ulcers. Inhalation of vesicant vapors causes shortness of breath, cough, wheezing, and pulmonary edema. Other nonspecific symptoms include nausea, vomiting and fatigue. Table 4-7 summarizes the signs and symptoms of vesicant agents.

The key difference between mustard agents and other vesicants is the onset of signs and symptoms. Lewisite and phosgene oxime cause immediate burning and pain to the skin, eyes, and respiratory tract. Exposed individuals will usually exit the area or don their protective masks and garments immediately upon exposure. This usually limits the total exposure of the patients and consequently limits injury.

In contrast, mustard agents cause no immediate symptoms on contact. Thus, individuals may not be aware of the exposure and fail to decontaminate or protect themselves from further exposure. Mustard exposure of only a few minutes will lead to

TABLE 4-7

SIGNS AND SYMPTOMS OF VESICANT AGENT EXPOSURE

Skin	burning, erythema, blistering
Eyes	stinging, tearing, ulcer formation, "blindness"
Respiratory	shortness of breath, cough, wheeze
Gastrointestinal	nausea and vomiting
Others	fatigue, lethargy

significant pain, redness, and blistering within two to twenty-four hours. Eye damage may occur earlier, often within one or two hours after exposure.

Severely exposed individuals may develop widespread skin and mucous membrane damage. Essentially, such patients have suffered large chemical burns. Pain, blindness, and respiratory distress will be prominent symptoms.

Emergency Care

The most important action when caring for a vesicant-exposed patient is immediate removal of the agent. The window of opportunity for preventing damage is only a few minutes. Immediate irrigation with water or a chemical decontamination kit is crucial. Since time is of the essence, this care must be provided by the patient himself or by a bystander. By the time the patient reaches the EMS provider, at least some damage has been done. Nonetheless, medical treatment includes continuing irrigation and decontamination. The type and amount of irrigation used will depend upon the available supply of water. Ideally, a hose (low pressure) provides plenty of water, but in even the small amount in a canteen is better than none. Saline from an IV bag is also useful, and is particularly suited for eye irrigation. Never delay irrigation of the eyes while searching for sterile saline. Use plain, uncontaminated water instead. Table 4-8 outlines the emergency care of vesicant agents.

TABLE 4-8

EMERGENCY TREATMENT OF VESICANT PATIENTS

IMMEDIATE TREATMENT	Copious irrigation and decontamination
MILD SKIN IRRITATION	Sterile dry dressing
SEVERE SKIN LESIONS, BLISTERS	Sterile dry dressing
SEVERE EYE LESIONS	Eye patch
SEVERE PAIN	Morphine IV
SEVERE RESPIRATORY DISTRESS	Oxygen, intubation if needed

Once blistering or other damage occurs, emergency care is the same as for ordinary chemical burns. Dry sterile dressings are applied loosely. Severe eye injuries should be patched. Most patients will be suffering significant pain and should receive intravenous morphine in 2 mg increments IV/IM. Unlike thermal burns, most serious vesicant patients do not require fluid resuscitation.

Triage and Decision Making

Most vesicant patients with less than 50% body surface area affected will be categorized as delayed. Over 50% body surface area affected would usually be considered expectant. This unfortunate patient could be saved, but only at the expense of great medical resources. Patients with eye involvement are considered delayed. Less than 5% body surface area affected are triaged minimal. Few vesicant patients will be triaged as immediate, except perhaps to institute irrigation, which should be part of self or bystander aid prior to reaching medical care.

CYANIDE

Overview

Cyanide is a rapidly acting lethal agent that directly poisons the body's cellular metabolism. It is the representative agent of what used to be termed "blood agents." This old term is a misnomer, since the site of action of cyanide is not the blood or red blood cells. Related chemicals with similar toxicities include hydrogen cyanide (AC), cyanogen chloride (CK), and cyanogen bromide. Although it is a potent poison, cyanide is 25-50 times less toxic by the inhalation route than the nerve agent GB (sarin). This limits its military usefulness. Cyanide is relatively easy and inexpensive to produce, and hence may represent a significant terrorist threat.

Cyanide was used in large quantities by the French in WWI, but its military effectiveness was limited. Japan allegedly used cyanide against China in WWII, and Iraq may have used the agent against the Kurds in the 1980s. The high volatility of cyanide means that it quickly evaporates and disperses. Thus, it is likely to affect only those individuals in the immediate area at the time of a cyanide release. An important exception might be a closed-space release, such as in a building. In this case, the enclosed space would slow the dispersion.

Cyanide exposure risk is not limited to chemical warfare and terrorist attacks. Thousands of tons of commercial cyanide and related compounds are manufactured and transported across the U.S. and other countries every year. Combustion of plastics, as in a structure fire, can also produce cyanide. Thus, all EMS providers must be familiar with the management of cyanide-poisoned patients.

Toxicity

Cyanide is usually absorbed by inhaling the vapor, however poisoning can also occur by ingesting cyanide-contaminated food or water. Once in the body, cyanide acts rapidly. If a large concentration is inhaled, loss of consciousness occurs within 1 minute and death within six to eight minutes. Moderate exposure will also produce unconsciousness and death, but there is sufficient time in which the EMS provider can act. Low dose exposures can make the patient briefly ill, but most will recover without treatment. This "all or nothing" phenomena of cyanide has important implications for treatment and triage as will be discussed.

Cyanide rapidly inactivates a metabolic enzyme called cytochrome a3. This enzyme is critical to all cells in the body, and it allows the utilization of oxygen for cellular energy. When cytochrome a3 is inactivated by cyanide, the cell immediately starves for oxygen and begins to die. No amount of supplemental oxygen can overcome this process (yet supplemental oxygen is still important to maximize oxygen delivery to those cells not yet poisoned by cyanide). The body can rid itself of small amounts of cyanide, and this accounts for the spontaneous recovery of patients with minimal exposures. Larger exposures overwhelm the body's natural cyanide detoxification, and unless treatment is promptly started, the patient will likely die.

Assessment

Cyanide works rapidly and primarily targets the brain and heart. Within a minute of inhaling a high concentration of cyanide, the victim loses consciousness and may convulse (seize). Two or three minutes later, the patient stops breathing. Cardiac arrest occurs within six to eight minutes of exposure.

Lower concentrations or ingestion of cyanide produces milder symptoms and a slower rate of onset. Anxiety, weakness, dizziness, nausea, and muscular trembling are common. Physical findings are nonspecific and may include elevated heart and respiratory rate. It is possible for symptoms to progress to loss of consciousness, apnea, and death. The "cherry red" color of the lips and extremities classically associated with cyanide poisoning is unreliable. The patient may be pale, cyanotic or normal color. The pulse oximeter may give a false sense of reassurance in cyanide poisoning. Although the blood may be well saturated with oxygen, cyanide causes cellular hypoxia by blocking the utilization of oxygen. Table 4-9 outlines the signs and symptoms of cyanide poisoning.

TABLE 4-9

SIGNS AND SYMPTOMS OF CYANIDE POISONING

HIGH CONCENTRATION - INHALED	30-60 sec loss of consciousness, convulsions two to three min apnea six to eight min cardiac arrest
INGESTION OR LOW CONCENTRATION INHALED	tachycardia tachypnea dizziness nausea weakness may progress to LOC, apnea and death

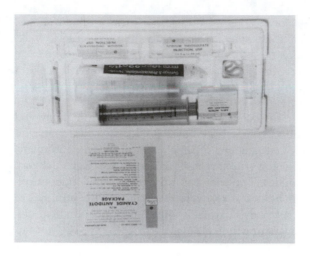

Figure 4-4 Cyanide antidote kit.

Emergency Care

To be effective, treatment of cyanide poisoning must be started early. Serious vapor exposures will result in severe respiratory distress or apnea in addition to unconsciousness. Rapid airway intervention (endotracheal intubation, if available) and ventilatory support with a bag-valve-mask is indicated as a first priority. However, a rapid shift to antidotal therapy will be required to save the patient.

The antidote for cyanide is a two-stage process using a nitrite compound followed by a sulfur-containing compound (Figure 4-4). The nitrite acts by converting the hemoglobin (the primary oxygen-carrying protein in the blood) in the blood to methemoglobin. Methemoglobin then binds the cyanide, removing it from the cytochrome a3. The sulfur-containing antidote then removes the cyanide by forming a nontoxic compound which is excreted in the urine. This process is depicted in Figure 4-5.

The nitrites for clinical use are sodium nitrite and amyl nitrite. If an IV is already established, administer sodium nitrite 300 mg (6-10 mg/kg up to 300 mg) over two to

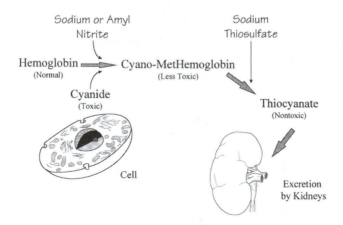

Figure 4-5 Removal of cyanide from cytochrome a_3 by use of nitrite and sulfur-containing antidotes.

TABLE 4-10

ADULT DOSE AND ADMINISTRATION OF CYANIDE ANTIDOTES
SEE TEXT FOR PEDIATRIC DOSES.

ANTIDOTE	DOSE	ROUTE	COMMENTS
Oxygen	high flow	mon-rebreather, BVM	Ventilatory support may be needed
Amyl nitrite	1 ampule	inhaled	Only if no IV access
Sodium nitrite	300 mg	IV	primary antidote
Sodium thiosulfate	12.5 gm	IV	Use only after sodium nitrite is given

four minutes. Amyl nitrite is used only when an IV is not yet established. Crush one ampule for the patient to inhale. If the patient has spontaneous respirations, place the ampule under an oxygen mask with high flow O2 running. In patients needing ventilatory support, place it in the bag or oxygen reservoir of the bag-valve mask. In all cases, be certain to avoid letting the ampule fall into the patient's mouth or down the ET tube. Always follow inhaled amyl nitrate with intravenous sodium nitrite. Do not use amyl nitrite if the patient has already received sodium nitrite.

Following administration of IV sodium nitrite, administer 12.5 gms (250-400 mg/kg up to 12.5 gm) of sodium thiosulfate. Use 5 ml of sodium thiosulfate for each ml of sodium nitrite. Do not use sodium thiosulfate unless the patient has received IV sodium nitrite, since it does not work well by itself. Table 4-10 outlines the dose and administration of cyanide antidotes. A highly effective and much safer antidote (related to vitamin B_{12}) is on the horizon, but is not yet available for general use in the US.

Triage and Decision Making

Patients with severe or progressing symptoms should be triaged as immediate patients. Patients who are pulseless are expectant. Those patients with mild, nonprogressing symptoms would be considered delayed or minimal depending on the severity of symptoms. Ambulatory patients, for example, would likely be minimal. In fact, if most symptoms resolve, these patients require no further emergent treatment.

The key decision facing the EMS provider when confronted with a potential cyanide poisoning is not triage, however. The hardest decision is whether to initiate antidotal therapy when hard evidence of cyanide poisoning is not present. Since the window of opportunity in treating cyanide poisoning is brief, the EMS provider must decide with whatever information is at hand. Certainly, if intelligence reports or chemical detection equipment indicates the presence of cyanide, the EMS provider should treat any patient with compatible signs and symptoms (Table 4-9) with antidotes.

Treatment with nitrites is not without side effects and risks. Hypotension and hypoxemia are possible effects. Keeping the patient supine (lying down) and providing supplemental oxygen will minimize these adverse effects.

PULMONARY AGENTS

Overview

Pulmonary agents include phosgene (CG), other halogen compounds, and various nitrogen-oxygen compounds. These agents act primarily to cause lung injury, hence the obsolete term "choking" agents. In WWI, both Germany and Britain used phosgene, usually in combination with chlorine, another pulmonary agent. Currently, phosgene and related agents are not considered very suitable for military use. However, the widespread availability of phosgene makes it a potential weapon for terrorists.

Over one billion pounds of phosgene are produced by industry in the U.S. for chemical processes. Millions of tons of chlorine ar produced and widely shipped in large containers. Pulmonary agents can be incidentally produced during combustion of plastics (particularly Teflon, or polytetrafluoroethylene) or munitions, including smoke (HC). Thus the EMS provider has ample opportunity to encounter pulmonary agents in the field.

Phosgene is the representative agent in this group, and the remainder of this section will focus on it. Phosgene is transported as a liquid, but it rapidly converts into a gas that tends to settle in low-lying locations. It has the odor of newly mown hay. The other pulmonary agents share similar properties and give similar symptoms. Emergency treatment for all agents in this class is the same.

Toxicity

Phosgene works by directly attacking the airway and lung tissue. The smaller airways and alveoli are most susceptible. The damaged airways and alveoli leak fluid, which leads to

---

TABLE 4-11

TREATMENT OF PHOSGENE OR PULMONARY AGENT EXPOSURE

MILD SYMPTOMS	beta-agonist nebulized (Albuterol)
Mild dyspnea	oxygen
Wheezing	rest
Cough	
SEVERE SYMPTOMS	
	above, plus
pulmonary edema	airway management
severe dyspnea	positive pressure ventilation
stridor	
airway obstruction	

---

pulmonary edema and inflammation. This, of course, causes dyspnea, hypoxemia and, if severe enough, respiratory failure.

Assessment

Relatively low concentrations of phosgene irritate the mucous membranes (mouth, eyes, nose, and throat) so initial symptoms will reflect tearing, runny nose and throat irritation. If the patient is exposed to a higher concentration, airway and lung damage may also occur. However, symptoms of pulmonary edema will take several hours. Thus a key point in dealing with phosgene patients is realizing that initially mild symptoms may lead to a serious condition within a few hours. Table 4-11 summarizes the signs and symptoms of phosgene inhalation. Exertion can worsen symptoms.

Emergency Care

Initial care of phosgene inhalation is the same as for other toxic inhalations. Priority is given to airway and breathing concerns. Mild to moderately symptomatic patients are treated with high flow oxygen and rest. Severe dyspnea may require airway control to include intubation. Signs of airway compromise, including obstruction and stridor, mandate immediate intubation. In extreme cases, needle cricothyrostomy or cricothyrotomy may be lifesaving.

Rest is an important component in the field treatment of phosgene exposure. Exertion or exercise worsens the symptoms of the exposure. Therefore, all patients with moderate to severe symptoms should not be allowed to ambulate unless absolutely necessary. The delayed effects of phosgene require that all exposed individuals undergo a period of observation for signs of worsening. Twenty-four hours is optimal, but even three to six hours of observation will be helpful in identifying progressing cases.

Patients exhibiting copious secretions will require suctioning. Shortness of breath, wheezing, tachypnea or muscular retractions should all be treated with a beta-2 agonist such as albuterol. The beta-2 agonist can be administered by inhalation by using a mouthpiece, mask, or endotracheal tube. A typical regimen might be 0.5 ml of albuterol solution dissolved in 5 ml normal saline administered by nebulization. The pediatric dose is 0.01 ml/kg. This treatment may be repeated every twenty minutes up to three times. This regimen may need to be repeated every three to four hours during long transports. No significant interval changes are required for pediatric patients. Table 4-11 summarizes treatment.

Triage and Decision Making

Patients suffering severe dyspnea, stridor or pulmonary edema require immediate field treatment to survive and are triaged as immediate. Patients with shortness of breath but no tachypnea, wheezing, crackles, or stridor are delayed. A patient with a known exposure but little or no signs or symptoms can be classified as minimal. These latter two categories must be rested and should be observed and reclassified, if necessary. Expectant patients manifest with signs of severe pulmonary edema (severe dyspnea, hypoxemia, crackles, muscular retractions, altered mental status) and hypotension. Even with intensive treatment, many of these patients will not survive.

Overview

Riot control agents include the common terms "tear gas" and "mace." Specific agents include CS, CN, CA, CR, and pepper spray (oleoresin capsicum, OC). Their common effect is intense irritation of the eyes, nose, and other mucous membranes. In the concentrations employed for field use, these agents are all considered non-lethal.

Agents in use today by US military and police forces are limited to CS, CN (mace), and pepper spray. The last agent has gained widespread acceptance as a safe agent for use in direct employment against individual suspects by civilian police. Thus all EMS providers must be familiar with these agents.

With the exception of pepper spray, all riot control agents are solids. The dispersion method aerosolizes the solid, which is seen as a white or gray cloud of "gas." Each of these agents causes pain without tissue damage. At extremely high concentrations (a closed room, for example or very close range), it is possible for these agents to have serious effects.

Assessment

Severe eye pain and tearing are characteristic of riot agents and lead to a temporary "blinding" of exposed individuals. Additionally, nose, throat, and skin irritation are also common. Cough and shortness of breath can also occur. In rare cases, wheezing, and bronchospasm may occur. Riot control agents, by design, give only temporary symptoms. Once in fresh air, exposed individuals will feel relief within fifteen minutes. Mild lingering effects may last for hours. Table 4-12 outlines the signs and symptoms of riot agents.

Emergency Care

Under most field conditions, emergency care is limited to removal of the patient to fresh air. The effects of riot control agents are self-limited and no further treatment is usually needed. On occasion, a patient may experience severe shortness of breath and wheezing. This should be treated with beta-2 agonists. It is possible that a patient close to the dispersion or detonation of the riot control agent may have a particle lodged in the eye.

TABLE 4-12

SIGNS AND SYMPTOMS OF RIOT AGENT EXPOSURES

Tearing and eye pain
Temporary "blindness"
Nose, throat and skin irritation
Coughing and shortness of breath

Treatment in this case involves copious irrigation with saline, ringers lactate, or plain water. Commercial products are available to treat the effects of riot control agents, but are not necessary since these agents cause only limited effects.

Triage and Decision Making

Since most patients will recover spontaneously, triage and emergency care are not needed. Those few patients with severe or persistent symptoms should be triaged in accordance with their symptoms.

Conclusion

With proper training and equipment, it is possible to provide advanced-level emergency care to patients of chemical agents. Knowledge of symptoms, signs, specific management and antidote treatments is critical for optimal chemical patient care.

FOR FURTHER READING

Medical Management of Chemical Patients, 2d ed. U.S. Army Medical Research Institute of Chemical Defense, Aberdeen Proving Grounds, MD. 1995

Field Manual 3-5 NBC Decontamination. Department of the Army, Washington, DC, 1993

Field Manual 3-4 NBC Protection. Department of the Army, Washington, DC 1992

Field Manual 8-285, Treatment of Chemical Agent Patients and Conventional Military Chemical Patients. Department of the Army, Washington, DC, 1995

Field Manual 8-9, NATO Handbook on Medical Aspects of NBC Defensive Operations. Department of the Army, Washington, DC, 1996

Emergency Response to Terrorism: Basic Concepts Student Manual. US Fire Administration, National Fire Academy. Emmitsburg, MD, 1997

MCCAUGHEY BG, et al: Combat casualties in conventional and chemical warfare environment. Military Medicine 1988; 153: 227-229

DANON YL, et al (eds): Chemical Warfare Medicine. Gefen Publishing House, Ltd. Jerusalem, 1994

SPIERS EM: Chemical and Biological Weapons. St. Martin's Press. New York, 1984

ZAJTCHUK R, et al (eds): Medical Aspects of Chemical and Biological Warfare. Department of the Army, Office of the Surgeon General, Washington, DC, 1997

BORAK J, et al: Hazardous Materials Exposure. Prentice-Hall, Englewood Cliffs, NJ, 1991

5

CARE OF BIOLOGICAL AGENT ILLNESSES

INTRODUCTION

Overview

Biological weapons are living organisms (or the toxins produced by living organisms) deliberately used to cause disease in the target population. Biological weapons are generally no different than the naturally occurring disease except that they are concentrated and delivered with the intent to cause harm.

Because a small amount of agent can cause widespread casualties, biological weapons are potential weapons of mass destruction. Because they cause disease that is identical to naturally occurring disease, it can be difficult (at least initially) to detect and identify the attack. The potential spread or contagiousness of many biological agents adds a new dimension to the threat and fear associated with weapons of mass destruction.

This chapter will review the principles of biological weapons and discuss a few types of agents. Identification and treatment priorities will be highlighted, along with the isolation measures needed to safely care for victims of biological agents.

History

Crude forms of biological warfare date as far back as the 14th to 18th centuries when attackers were known to hurl the corpses of bubonic plague victims over the walls of besieged cities. In the 1750s, the English "donated" smallpox-laden blankets to Indians loyal to the French in the French and Indian War. This caused many casualties among the native Americans fighting alongside the French.

In WWII, the Japanese in particular had an active biological weapons program. After the war and until 1972, the U.S. manufactured and stockpiled a number of agents.

Since 1972, international treaty has banned the development or use of biological weapons, but several nations are still believed to posses offensive biological agents. These nations include Iraq and several republics of the former Soviet Union.

Current Threat

Today the threat of biological attack is believed to be higher than in the past. Several countries with terrorist tendencies continue to experiment with these agents. Because of the difficulty in tracing an attack, terrorist groups may find biological agents useful tools in carrying out their deadly work. For this reason, all prehospital providers must be knowledgeable and skilled in dealing with this potential threat.

NATURE OF BIOLOGICAL AGENTS

Biological agents for warfare or terrorism are simply disease-causing organisms (or the products of organisms) that are collected, processed and delivered for maximal effect, usually death. Any of the disease-forming groups such as viruses, bacteria, or fungus are potential candidates. Fortunately, weapons-makers have only a few options to choose from, because an agent must be effective, easily delivered, and easy to manufacture. This limits the list of potential agents, and the EMS provider can train to care for this small number of biological agents. Table 1-5 (chapter 1, Medical Aspects of WMD) outlines some important characteristics of biological agents.

Delivery

To be effective, the biological agent must get to its target. This is usually accomplished by spraying a liquid containing the agent through a nozzle. A nozzle attached to an airplane could deliver the agent over a wide area. A particle size of 1-5 microns is optimal because it has the greatest chance of dispersing and also of reaching deep into the respiratory tract, the most effective portal of entry. Wind speed and direction, rain, and sunlight can each have a great effect on delivery. High winds will tend to disperse the agent but can also carry it great distances. Rain and sunshine usually work to diminish the agent's effectiveness. Ideal conditions for the release of biological agents usually occur at night and very early in the morning.

Route of Exposure

By far, the respiratory tract is the most common and efficient portal of entry for most biological agents. Particle size is important (Figure 5-1). If the particle is too big (> 5 microns), it will impact in the upper respiratory tract and be less effective. If it is too small (< 1 micron) it will not impact in the lungs but will merely be exhaled back out. Lesser portals include the mouth, nose, and eye mucous membranes. Ingestion of the biological agent is a serious consideration if the attacker contaminates the food or water supply.

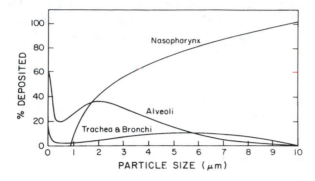

Figure 5-1 Particle size is important to deposition in the respiratory tract.

Disease States

Most biological warfare agents are intended to kill their victims. Anthrax, botulinum toxin and tularemia are examples of lethal agents. Other agents tend to incapacitate, such as Q fever and staphylococcal enterotoxin B. The actual disease state varies with each agent. Plague and Q fever cause a pneumonia-like picture of cough, fever, and shortness of breath. Cholera, on the other hand produces vomiting and diarrhea.

Lethality

Biological agents can be extremely potent weapons. Some of the most toxic substances known to man are potential biological weapons. Table 5-1 lists the toxicity of several biological agents as compared to other poisons. For example, 50 kg of anthrax dispersed upwind of a large city could kill up to 220,000 people. Thus, the potential power of biological weapons should not be underestimated.

TABLE 5-1

TOXICITY OF SOME BIOLOGICAL AGENTS AND OTHER POISONS

AGENT	LETHAL DOSE UG/KG	LETHAL DOSE 70 KG ADULT
Botulinum toxin	0.001	0.07 ug
Ricin	3.0	210 ug
VX nerve agent	15.0	1 mg
SEB	27.0	2 mg
Sarin (GB)	100	7 mg
T2 mycotoxin	1,210	85 mg

Adapted from Medical Management of Biological Casualties, 2d ED, U.S. Army
Research Institute of Infectious Diseases, Ft Detrick, MD 1996

Recognition of Attack

Key to distinguishing a biological attack from an isolated case of ordinary (or perhaps exotic) disease is the number and timing of cases. Isolated disease strikes one or at most a few persons. If cases are contagious (like the common cold) more may become infected, but only over time. Biological attacks, in contrast, usually strike a large number of individuals at virtually the same time. Symptoms all develop within hours, or at most days of each other. This situation is easily distinguishable from isolated cases.

A little more challenging is differentiating a biological attack from ordinary mass food poisoning or perhaps epidemic meningitis. The key here is to recognize the common bond shared by all the ill patients—a shared meal, water source, or living quarters. Biological attacks usually strike victims across large areas without regards to job, residence, meal source, or similar factors.

SPECIFIC AGENTS

There are about a dozen biological agents which are sufficiently threatening to warrant discussion. They can be roughly divided into four groups: 1) pneumonia-like agents, 2) encephalitis-like agents, 3) biological toxins, and 4) other agents. While these groupings are artificial, they are useful to the EMS provider who must recognize and treat biological patients without the benefit of extensive experience in exotic infectious diagnosis and sophisticated laboratory support.

Treatment

Effective treatment of biological agents requires accurate identification (diagnosis) of the offending agent. This can be quite challenging in the field since rapid field laboratory analysis is as yet unavailable. Instead, EMS providers must rely on intelligence reports and history and physical examination to identify the likely cause. In this chapter specific antiobiotic and antitoxin treatments are outlined. It is expected that the EMS provider will work closely with medical direction when considering these treatnment modalities.

Pneumonia-like Agents

This group (Table 5-2) includes anthrax, tularemia, plague, and Q fever. Common symptoms include cough, dyspnea, fever and malaise. Anthrax is by far the most lethal, infecting and killing up to half the exposed persons. Q-fever, on the other hand, is an incapacitating agent and rarely causes death. In general, these are the agents most likely to be used in a biological weapon.

Anthrax

Anthrax is caused by the bacterium Bacillus anthracis and in nature usually infects cattle, sheep and horses. The handling of meat, bone meal and hides of these animals can pass the disease to humans, usually through direct contact. The bacteria can also form

TABLE 5-2

BIOLOGICAL AGENTS CAUSING PNEUMONIA-LIKE ILLNESS

AGENT	COMMON SYMPTOMS	SPECIFIC FINDINGS
Anthrax	Cough, shortness of breath, fever, malaise	Severe dyspnea, shock, death within twenty-four to thirty-six hours
Plague		headache, hemoptysis severe dyspnea, death
Q fever		resolves two to fourteen days
Tularemia		respirophasic chest pain, headache

spores, which are highly resistant to heat and drying and can be easily aerosolized. The spore is the usual infective form in biological weapons.

Several nations, including the US, the republics of the former Soviet Union, and Iraq are believed to have or be capable of making anthrax. Relatively speaking, it is easy to manufacture and store anthrax. Delivery, particularly over wide areas, is more difficult, but could be accomplished by aerosolization of the spores from aircraft or by detonating small bombs encased with anthrax spores.

Anthrax has a very high fatality rate; that is, 90% or more of those who contract the disease from inhaling the organism will die. After an incubation period of one to six days, a nonspecific illness of fever, malaise, nonproductive cough and chest discomfort will occur. In theory, persons aggressively treated at this stage may recover. Untreated, however, anthrax progresses to a brief (hours to days) period of improvement followed by the rapid appearance of respiratory distress and diaphoresis. The lesions and scabs characteristic of skin exposure may not occur from inhalational anthrax. Shock and death ensue within one to two days.

Treatment of anthrax requires aggressive respiratory and cardiovascular support. Oxygen and intubation will be required in many cases. Most will require intravenous fluids to counteract septic shock. Intravenous ciprofloxacin 400 mg every eight to twelve hours or doxycycline 100 mg every twelve hours are the antibiotics of choice. Children may be treated with penicillin up to two million units IV every 2 hours plus streptomycin IM 30 mg/kg/day in two divided doses or gentamycin IV 3-5 mg/kg/day. Despite aggressive therapy, many patients with pulmonary anthrax will die.

Prophylaxis is possible with a licensed vaccine that requires six initial doses over a year followed by yearly boosters. Vaccination may not entirely prevent disease but can provide reasonable protection. In the face of an imminent anthrax attack, ciprofloxacin 500 mg po bid or doxycycline 1000 mg po bid for adults may offer some protection. Contact isolation is required for infected patients. Hypochlorite solution effectively inactivates anthrax spores.

Plague

Plague is caused by the bacterium Yersinia pestis that naturally infects rodents such as mice, rats and squirrels in some parts of the world. Fleas that live on the rodents can occasionally pass the disease to humans. Crowded and unsanitary conditions can allow the disease to spread and accounts for the millions killed by plague in the European Middle Ages. Yersinia is quite hardy and can tolerate drying, freezing and heat well.

The most likely form of plague from a biological attack is pneumonic plague. This is usually caused by the inhalation of organisms, although it can occasionally occur from systemic spread through the blood. After an incubation period of two to three days, the victim develops high fever, chills, cough with hemoptysis (bloody sputum), headache and malaise. The pneumonia progresses rapidly and the patient soon develops cyanosis and shock. Death is from respiratory failure and septic shock. The black, necrotic skin lesions of cutaneous or bubonic plague are not usually seen in primary pneumonic plague. Approximately 100% of patients with pneumonic plague will die without treatment.

Treatment focuses on the respiratory and cardiovascular systems. Oxygen, intubation, mechanical ventilation and aggressive fluid resuscitation may all be required. If treatment with antibiotics is provided early in the course of the disease, recovery is possible. Intravenous doxycycline 100 mg every twelve hours or intramuscular streptomycin 30 mg/kg/day bid are the drugs of choice. Gentamycin 3-5 mg/kg/day IV may be substituted for streptomycin.

A licensed vaccine is available, but requires biannual boosters. Doxycycline 100 mg po bid is potentially effective in the face of imminent attack. Contact and respiratory isolation is required for pneumonic plague patients. Hypochlorite solution effectively destroys the plague bacterium.

Tularemia

Tularemia is caused by the bacterium Francisella tularensis and naturally infects rabbits. Humans can acquire the disease through handling infected materials or by the bites of deerflies, mosquitos and ticks. The bacterium is highly resistant to freezing but is susceptible to high heat. As few as 10 to 50 organisms can cause infection if inhaled.

Tularemia can appear in several forms in humans, depending on the route of exposure. Biological weapons will usually employ the aerosol route and cause typhoidal disease or pneumonia. Typical symptoms include fever, substernal chest discomfort and non-productive cough. Treatment includes respiratory and fluid support as needed and either streptomycin (30 mg/kg/day IM in two divided doses each day) or gentamycin (3-5 mg/kg/day IV). A vaccine is under development. Contact isolation is required for infected patients. Hypochlorite solution effectively kills F. tularnsis.

Q Fever

Q fever is caused by the rickettsial organism Coxiella burnetii. In nature, it infects sheep, cattle and goats. Humans may acquire the disease through aerosolization of infected urine, feces or milk. The organism is extremely potent: only a single inhaled organism may cause disease. Fortunately, Q fever is rarely fatal, and would thus be classified as an incapacitating agent.

Incubation lasts from 10 to 20 days, then victims develop symptoms lasting two days to two weeks. The usual symptoms are fever, myalgias (body aches), headache and malaise. Cough and respirophasic (pleuritic) chest pain can occur in about a fourth of cases. Complications can occur but are uncommon.

Treatment with oral tetracycline 500 mg qid or doxycycline 100 mg bid may shorten the course of the disease. Children should be treated with a macrolide antibiotic such as erythromycin. A vaccine is under development, but is not yet available. Prophylactic administration of oral tetracycline or doxycycline can prevent or delay the onset of disease. Standard body-fluid protection measures are adequate to protect health care workers and others. Hypochlorite solution effectively kills C. burnetii.

Encephalitis-Like Agents

Table 5-3 lists two agents that cause symptoms vaguely resembling those of influenza including fever, headache, and malaise. However, these diseases are many times more lethal than the flu. Their predilection for affecting the brain and central nervous system accounts for their rough classification as encephalitis agents. In this group, both the smallpox and Venezuelan equine encephalitis viruses have very high attack rates, affecting over 90% of those exposed. Both groups of agents can cause fatalities, with smallpox being the most deadly.

Smallpox

Smallpox is caused by the variola virus. Smallpox is believed to be eradicated from nature; however, laboratory repositories remain in the US and Russia. It is possible that other nations have secretly kept smallpox stocks. More than 30% of infected victims may die of the disease. Even vaccinated individuals may contract smallpox, and up to 3% will die.

Incubation lasts about twelve days, after which the patient develops abrupt fever, malaise, rigors, headache, backache and vomiting. About 15% will develop mental status changes (delirium). Two to three days later the characteristic rash appears on the face, hands and forearms. The rash spreads to the lower extremities, and finally begins to scab and heal in eight to fourteen days.

TABLE 5-3

BIOLOGICAL AGENTS CAUSING ENCEPHALITIS-LIKE ILLNESS

AGENT	COMMON SYMPTOMS	SPECIFIC FINDINGS
Small pox	Headache Fever Malaise	Characteristic rash develops in two to three days
Venezuelan Equine Encephalitis		severe headache photophobia

Treatment is supportive since antibiotics are ineffective against viruses. Respiratory and contact isolation are needed for infected patients. All unprotected contacts with an infected person should be quarantined for seventeen days. A licensed vaccine is available. Hypochlorite solution effectively inactivates the smallpox virus.

Venezuelan Equine Encephalitis

Venezuelan equine encephalitis (VEE) is caused by an alphavirus and is endemic to parts of Central and South America and Florida. As its name implies, horses, donkeys and mules are the natural reservoir. It is transmitted to humans by mosquitos. The attack rate of the disease is very high, approaching 90%. Fortunately, most recover and only 1% will die.

After a one to five day incubation period, the victim develops abrupt fever, chills, severe headache, photophobia, and myalgias. Nausea, vomiting and sore throat may also occur. The disease peaks for two to three days, then subsides. Malaise may last for one to two weeks. Complications include neurological problems such as brain damage. Children appear more susceptible to complications.

Treatment for VEE is supportive only. An experimental vaccine is under development. Infected patients require blood and body fluid precautions. Hypochlorite solution is effective against the VEE virus.

Miscellaneous Agents

Cholera, brucellosis and viral hemorrhagic fevers give signs and symptoms different from each other and from other agents discussed (Table 5-4). Viral hemorrhagic fevers include the infamous ebola virus and the agents of Dengue and yellow fever. These agents are lethal, causing death in 5-50% of infected individuals. Cholera is interesting because it is seen regularly in natural outbreaks and epidemics in developing nations. The watery diarrhea associated with it can be profuse and can easily dehydrate and kill a small child in less than one day or an adult in two or three days.

TABLE 5-4

MISCELLANEOUS BIOLOGICAL AGENTS

AGENT	SYMPTOMS AND FINDINGS
Cholera	Vomiting, abdominal distension profuse watery diarrhea severe dehydration possible
Viral Hemorrhagic Fevers	malaise, body aches, headache, vomiting, early easy bleeding, hypotension, shock late
Brucellosis	Fever, malaise, body aches, joint pain, headache, cough

Cholera

Cholera is caused by the Vibrio cholerae bacterium and naturally occurs in man. Transmission is by the "fecal-oral" route, that is, by eating or drinking contaminated food and water. The organism is very susceptible to drying, heat and water chlorination. It can live for days in untreated water, however.

Following an incubation period of twleve to seventy-two hours, victims experience sudden and uncomfortable abdominal cramping and a profuse, watery diarrhea. Vomiting and malaise may accompany the diarrhea. The diarrhea can result in the loss of five to ten liters of water per day and can easily lead to dehydration and hypovolemic shock. Death results from electrolyte imbalance and hypovolemia. Up to 50% of untreated victims will die. With adequate treatment, however, survival is excellent.

Treatment is aimed at preventing and correcting hypovolemic shock. Oral hydration with "World Health Organization oral rehydration solution" (contains water, sodium chloride, potassium chloride, sodium bicarbonate, and glucose) is frequently successful in adults and some children. Field expedient substitutes include juices and "sports drinks" such as Gatorade. Intravenous normal saline (preferably with bicarbonate and potassium added) can be lifesaving for seriously ill individuals. Children are much more susceptible to serious dehydration from cholera than are adults. Antibiotic treatment with tetracycline 500 mg qid or doxycycline 100 mg bid is frequently helpful. Resistant strains of cholera may require treatment with ciprofloxacin 500 mg bid or erythromycin 500 mg qid. Children should be treated with tetracycline 50 mg/kg/day qid for three days, erythromycin 40 mg/kg/day qid or trimethoprim-sulfamethoxazole 40 mg/kg/day bid, all for three days duration.

A vaccine is available but is only about 50% effective in preventing disease and requires a booster every six months. Since biological attacks must reach their victims through ingestion of the organism, the major mode of prevention is good sanitation. Careful protection of food and water sources, proper storage of foodstuffs, adequate water chlorination, and good handwashing technique will go a long way in preventing disease. Infected individuals require enteric precautions and all persons in contact should practice effective handwashing. Hypochlorite solution is extremely effective at destroying the cholera bacterium.

Brucellosis

Brucellosis is caused by the organism of the genus Brucella. This bacteria naturally infects sheep, pigs, goats, dogs and other mammals. Disease occurs in man from contact with infected animals or their milk. Brucella is highly infectious and can gain entry to the body through breaks in the skin, the mucous membranes, the lungs and the gastrointestinal tract. The most likely route for a biological attack would be by inhalation.

The signs and symptoms of brucellosis are nonspecific and can vary form person to person. The incubation period lasts from three days to three weeks. Fever, malaise, myalgias (body aches), sweats, and arthralgias (joint pain) are the most common symptoms. Cough and headache are also common, but these symptoms do not predominate. Untreated, the symptoms can last for weeks or months. Common complications include debilitating bone and joint disease. A rare complication is involvement of the heart called endocarditis, and this complication accounts for 80% of deaths from brucellosis.

Treatment is aimed at preventing and treating shock and cardiovascular collapse. Intravenous fluids will be necessary in severe cases. Endocarditis is a particularly feared complication as treatment of heart valve damage is difficult. Optimal treatment for adults is oral doxycycline 200 mg/day combined with oral rifampin 600-900 mg/day for six weeks. Trimethoprim-sulfamethoxazole may be substituted for the rifampin. Gentamycin may be substituted for streptomycin. Endocarditis or other serious complications may require triple antibiotic coverage including streptomycin or gentamycin for six weeks or longer.

Doxycycline and rifampin may be taken orally in combination for prophylaxis, but the effectiveness of this regimen is untested. There is no vaccine available. Infected patients require standard universal precautions. Hypochlorite solution effectively destroys the brucellosis bacterium.

Viral Hemorrhagic Fevers

Viral hemorrhagic fevers (VHF) include the deadly ebola and Marburg virus (Filoviridae), Lassa fever, Argentine hemorrhagic fever (Arenaviridae), hantavirus (Bunyaviridae), Rift Valley fever (Phleboviridae), and yellow and Dengue fever (Flaviviridae). This broad collection of viral diseases all have similar clinical features and are therefore considered together. Some, such as ebola and Marburg occur naturally in primates, including man. Argentine hemorrhagic fever occurs naturally in rodents and is spread by fecal matter. Yellow and Dengue fever are spread by mosquitos. All the VHFs (except Dengue virus) are infectious as aerosols and through direct contact with infectious material. Therefore, each has some potential as a biological weapon.

The incubation period for the VHFs is variable, but generally a few days to a week. Early symptoms include fever and malaise and early signs include conjunctival infection and petechia (tiny patches of bleeding in the skin). Full blown disease involves widespread damage to the capillary beds with easy bleeding, petechia, hypotension, and liver disease. Mortality can be in the range of 5-20%, with ebola causing death in 50-90% of those infected.

Treatment is supportive and includes judicious use of intravenous fluids. Overhydration is to be avoided, owing to the leaky capillary beds that may lead to pulmonary edema. Antibiotics are not helpful. However, the antiviral drug ribavirin has shown promise in treating some VHFs.

A yellow fever vaccine is available now and other VHF vaccines are under development. Barrier isolation (mask, gown and gloves) is required for all infected patients. VHF viruses can be present in high concentrations in the blood of infected patients, so careful handling of specimens and sharps is required. Hypochlorite solution effectively inactivates all the VHF viruses.

Biological Toxins

Biological toxins are perhaps the most significant threat of all the biological agents. Unlike anthrax, tularemia, and the other previously discussed agents, toxins are not living organisms. Instead, they are the products of living organisms. Therefore, toxins cannot be transmitted from an affected individual to another. This does not diminish the toxin threat, however, since biological toxins are among the most dangerous compounds

TABLE 5-5

CLINICAL EFFECTS OF BIOLOGICAL TOXINS

AGENT	EFFECTS
botulinum	generalized weakness and paralysis droopy eyelids, double vision, difficulty speaking, swallowing and breathing, respiratory failure and death
SEB	fever, chills headache body aches cough shock and death at high exposures
Ricin	Weakness fever cough hypotension and death
T2	pain, itching, redness and lesions on exposed skin nose and throat pain runny nose and sneezing shock and death at high exposures

known to man. By way of example, botulinum toxin is 15,000 times as potent as VX, the most deadly of all nerve agents.

There are dozens of potential biological toxins. Fortunately, only four are of significance: botulinum, ricin, staphylococcus enterotoxin 13 (SEB) and trichothecene mycotoxins (T2). Each gives varied effects (Table 5-5). Of particular importance is recognition of the paralysis and double vision (with normal mental status) of botulinum toxin and the skin lesions of T2.

Botulinum

Botulinum toxin is produced by the bacterium Clostridium botulinum and is the most toxic substance known to man. As little as 1 nanogram (1 billionth of a gram) per kilogram of botulinum will kill a man. This is a microscopic quantity! The route of exposure can either be inhalation or ingestion. A few sporadic cases of botulinum poisoning occur in the US each year, mostly from improperly canned food. Botulinum toxin is very stable and resists heat and freezing. Hypochlorite solution effectively inactivates the toxin. Because of its incredible potency and relative ease of manufacture, botulinum is considered a likely biological weapon threat.

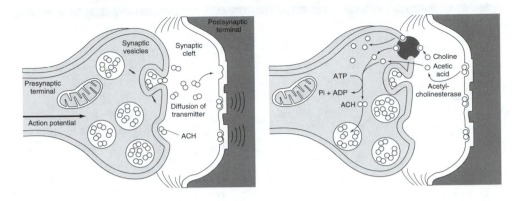

Figure 5-2 Presynaptic nerve ending at the neuromuscular junction. Normally, Acetylcholine is released and stimulates the muscle. Botulinum blocks this release and prevents stimulation.

Botulinum toxin acts by permanently binding to the presynaptic terminal of the neuromuscular junction (Figure 5-2). This inhibits nerve transmission and results in widespread muscular weakness and paralysis. Essentially, the nerve cannot release the neurotransmitter acetylcholine (ACh), and thus cannot stimulate the muscle. This may be thought of as the opposite effect of nerve agent poisoning, which causes an excess of ACh. The net effect of botulinum toxicity is complete paralysis, including the respiratory muscles, yet preservation of cardiac and higher mental functions. Untreated, foodborne botulism kills 60% of victims. Weaponized botulinum may kill an even higher percentage of victims.

As soon as twenty-four to thirty-six hours after ingestion or inhalation, victims experience blurred vision, dry mouth and difficulty talking and swallowing. A characteristic symptom is double vision (diplopia) and a useful sign is dilated pupils (mydriasis). A short time later, muscular weakness and paralysis sets in, which may eventually lead to respiratory arrest. Fever is absent and mental status is preserved (unless the patient is hypoxic from respiratory failure).

It is important to distinguish botulinum toxicity from nerve agent poisoning and atropine overdose (Table 5-6). This is important for rescuers and patients who may have received atropine for presumed nerve agent poisoning. Military experience shows that in the early stages of a chemical or biological attack, symptoms can be vague or confusing, leading to the use of atropine. The atropine itself causes symptoms, adding to the confusion.

Treatment focuses on respiratory support. Oxygen, intubation and mechanical ventilation can be lifesaving. Complete recovery from even severe botulinum toxicity is possible if respiratory support is initiated and continued until recovery (which can take weeks). This aggressive approach is not practical in a mass casualty situation, but is completely reasonable if only a few patients are encountered. Antitoxin therapy is an important adjunct to airway and breathing support. The antitoxin will neutralize any circulating botulinum toxin in the blood, but cannot reverse any toxin already bound to the nerve endings. In adults, 10 ml is administered intravenously over twenty minutes. Because the antitoxin can cause life-threatening anaphylaxis as well as other serious side effects, it may require skin testing and should be administered only by medical personnel familiar with its use.

TABLE 5-6

DIFFERENTIATING NERVE AGENT, BOTULINUM AND ATROPINE POISONING

FACTOR	NERVE AGENT	BOTULINUM	ATROPINE OVERDOSE
Time of Onset	Minutes	Hours	Minutes
Mental Status	Normal Initially Unconscious Late	Normal (Delirium)	Altered
Pupils	Miosis (Constricted)	Mydriasis (Dilated)	Mydriasis (Dilated)
Vision	Blurred	Often Double (Diplopia)	Blurred
Heart Rate	Decreased (Bradycardia)	Normal (Tachycardia)	Increased
Skin	Moist	Dry	Dry
Muscle Tone	Fasciculations Early Seizures Late	Progressive Flaccid Paralysis	Normal
Secretions	Copious	Normal	Dry
Small Airways	Bronchoconstriction	Normal	Bronchodilation

An experimental vaccine is being developed against botulinum toxin. It often causes uncomfortable local reactions and requires boosters each year. Botilinum-intoxicated patients are not able to transmit the disease and no special isolation measures (beyond universal precautions) are required.

Staphylococcal Enterotoxin B

Staphylococcal enterotoxin B (SEB) is produced by the common bacterium Staphylococcus aureus. This is one of the toxins that can cause ordinary food poisoning. SEB can enter the body through the inhalational or oral route, and produces differing clinical pictures depending on which route. The toxin is resistant to heat and only tiny quantities are needed to produce symptoms. Under most circumstances, SEB is not lethal, but can effectively incapacitate at least 50% of those exposed.

Approximately three to twelve hours after inhalation, SEB causes fever, chills, body aches and nonproductive cough. Shortness of breath and chest pain are possible. The fever may last for five days and the cough for up to a month. Ingested SEB produces severe nausea and vomiting and occasionally diarrhea. It is possible to have patients with overlapping symptoms since some aerosolized SEB may land on the hands or on food and be inadvertently swallowed by the victim.

Treatment is supportive, since there is no known antidote or effective treatment. Patients with dyspnea should receive oxygen, and hypotension and dehydration should be treated with intravenous saline fluid boluses. Except in cases of overwhelming toxicity, recovery is the rule. There is no known prophylaxis. Hypochlorite solution effectively inactivates the toxin when applied to most nonporous surfaces.

Ricin

Ricin is derived from the beans of the castor plant (Ricinus communis) which is grown worldwide. Ricin is a natural byproduct of castor oil production, making the acquisition of large quantities of the toxin relatively easy. The toxin may be either inhaled or ingested. It is a protein complex, and thus is susceptible to heat and weak hypochlorite solutions.

Ricin exerts its toxicity directly on cells by inhibiting protein synthesis. This causes cellular death and tissue necrosis. The aerosol route causes primary lung damage, pulmonary edema, respiratory distress and hypoxia. Ingested ricin causes severe vomiting, diarrhea, abdominal cramping and shock. Complications of ricin poisoning include multiple organ failure and disseminated intravascular coagulation.

After a latent period of about eight hours, aerosol-exposed individuals experience dyspnea, chest tightness, cough, fever, malaise and body aches (myalgias). Death occurs within thirty-six to seventy-two hours from pulmonary edema and respiratory failure.

Treatment is supportive as there is no known antitoxin. Respiratory failure is treated with oxygen, and if needed, intubation and mechanical ventilation. Hypotension and shock will require intravenous fluids. There is currently no vaccine available. Ricin-intoxicated individuals require no special isolation or precautions once they have had effective skin decontamination. Hypochlorite solution effectively denatures ricin, rendering it ineffective.

Trichothecene Mycotoxins

Trichothecene mycotoxins (T2) are the products of fungus molds fusarium, trichoderma, myrotecium, stachybotrys, and others. These are the alleged toxins of "yellow rain" in Laos, Kampuchea, and Afghanistan. Given its appearance in several global locations over time, T2 should be considered a potential biological weapon.

T2 acts directly on cellular growth by inhibiting protein and nucleic acid synthesis. Rapidly dividing cells are most affected, accounting for the symptoms referable to the skin, mucous membranes, gastrointestinal tract and bone marrow. In a biological attack, exposure is possible through inhalation, contact and oral routes. This will produce broad array of effects on the victim. The toxin is very stable even under high heat and prolonged sunlight.

T2 acts almost immediately, causing symptoms within minutes to hours of exposure. Burning skin, redness, pain, blistering and bleeding at exposed skin sites occurs. Contact with the upper respiratory tract causes nose and throat pain, rhinorrhea (nasal discharge) and nosebleed (epistaxis). Lower respiratory symptoms include dyspnea, wheezing and hemoptysis (bloody sputum). Eye exposure causes redness, pain, tearing and blurry vision. Gastrointestinal exposure results in nausea, vomiting, bloody diarrhea and abdominal cramping. Significant exposure can result in dizziness, loss of balance and coordination, hypotension and death.

T2 exposure can be hard to differentiate from mustard agent poisoning. However, mustard agents have a characteristic odor and are readily detected by field tests. Mustard usually has a slower onset of action, taking several hours to produce symptoms.

There is no specific therapy for T2 mycotoxins. Medical management should focus on thorough decontamination (hypochlorite solution is effective). Saline should be used to decontaminate the eyes. Respiratory distress should be treated with oxygen,

TABLE 5-7

PRINCIPLES OF EMERGENCY CARE FOR BIOLOGICAL AGENT PATIENTS

Recognition and identification
Isolation in selected cases
Respiratory and fluid support as needed
Arrange antibiotic or antitoxin therapy

aerosolized beta-agonists (albuterol), and if necessary, intubation and mechanical ventilation. Skin lesions should be dressed with dry gauze. Hypotension and shock are treated with intravenous fluids such as saline. There is no vaccine or prophylaxis available. Decontaminated patients require no special isolation or precautions.

EMERGENCY CARE

Recognition and Identification

A number of principles are important when faced with a biological patient (Table 5-7). Recognition is crucial to the successful management of biological patients. By the very nature of biological attacks, many patients can be expected and the EMS provider will need to call additional resources as early as possible. A top priority is self protection. Physicians (or physician assistants) will be needed to prescribe the proper antibiotic coverage and antitoxin treatment so crucial in treating biological agents. Infectious disease and biological agent experts and laboratory support will also be needed to help positively identify the agent and recommend further treatment. Field laboratory identification is not currently possible but a number of research initiatives are working to solve this problem.

Isolation

Only a few biological agents are highly contagious from one infected individual to another. In particular, smallpox, plague, and ebola are highly transmissible. As much as practical in the field, isolate biological patients from unaffected individuals. Enforce the protective measures outlined in this chapter (Figure 5-3). Once the agent is identified as non transmissible, overt protection can be discontinued. In all situations of patient care, observe universal precautions if contact with body fluids is likely.

Supportive Care

The usual principles of emergency care apply to the care of biological patients. Priority goes to securing and maintaining an airway and ensuring adequate ventilation. Provide high flow oxygen by non rebreather mask to all patients in moderate to severe respiratory distress. Respiratory failure or apnea will necessitate orotracheal intubation or positive

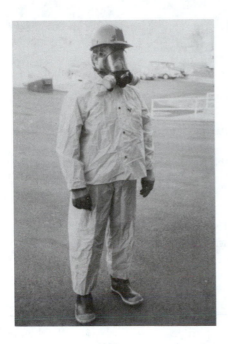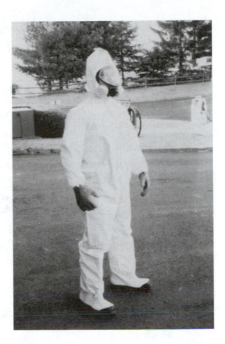

Figure 5-3 Personal protective equipment consisting of a filtration respirator, head and face protection, impervious boots and gloves and body splash protection is adequate for most biological agents.

pressure ventilation with a bag-valve mask. Respiratory support is particularly crucial in botulinum poisoning. The cause of death in botulinum poisoning is respiratory failure. If ventilation can be maintained for the patient, the chance of survival is good. Continued ventilation in the hospital may be necessary for weeks or months.

Intravenous lifelines or saline locks should be initiated on all nonambulatory biological patients. Many agents will cause dehydration, hypotension or septic shock, and thus early IV access is important. Adult patients with signs of compensated shock should receive an initial 1,000 ml of normal saline as a bolus. Children should receive 20 ml/kg. Uncompensated shock (e.g., hypotension or signs of inadequate perfusion) should receive repeat boluses up to 3,000 ml for adults or 60 ml/kg for children. During prolonged transportation patients may receive up to 1,000 ml (20 ml/kg) every two hours as a bolus if signs of shock persist.

Antibiotic and Antitoxin Therapy

A mainstay of treatment for many biological agents is use of specific antibiotics or antitoxins. These treatments require the expertise of a physician or PA in selecting the right drug, dose, and route. It is beyond the scope of practice and beyond the expectations of EMS providers to initiate this therapy. The EMS provider does play a crucial role in summoning the assistance of a physician when necessary, and can assist the physician's treatment of biological patients with antibiotics or antitoxins. For purposes of familiarization, some antibiotics and antitoxins are mentioned in this chapter. Selection and use of these medications is best left to a physician.

Immunization and Prophylaxis

Perhaps the best protection against biological weapons is prevention. A key tool for prevention of any disease is immunization or prophylaxis. Immunization involves taking substances related to the biological agent (but nontoxic and noninfectious) to develop resistance or antibodies. Immunizations are available against many biological agent threats. Prophylaxis is the taking of antibiotics prior to exposure or during the incubation stage. Some sort of advanced warning or good intelligence report is needed to pinpoint the agent and timing of an attack to make this strategy useful. Several effective immunizations and prophylaxis strategies are available. The most notable is the anthrax vaccine, which may be up to 95% effective and is relatively free of side effects. Other immunizations and prophylactic antibiotics are administered only when the threat is high. Table 5-8 lists several common preventive strategies against biological agents.

TRIAGE AND DECISION MAKING

Triage for biological patients is no different than triage of any other patient. By the very nature of biological attacks, the EMS provider will likely face mass casualties. In general, ambulatory patients will be classified as minimal, while those with moderate to severe symptoms (severe headache, cough, malaise, vomiting, etc.) and those unable to walk would be considered delayed. Patients requiring immediate respiratory support with positive pressure ventilation and those in uncompensated shock are immediate. Pulseless patients and those with persistent uncompensated shock despite initial IV fluid boluses are generally considered expectant. Table 5-9 summarizes the triage decision-making of biological mass casualty incidents.

TABLE 5-8

IMMUNIZATION AND PROPHYLAXIS STRATEGIES
FOR SOME POTENTIAL BIOLOGICAL AGENTS

AGENT	STRATEGY
Anthrax	Vaccine, or ciprofloxacin/doxycycline prophylaxis
Plague	Vaccine, or doxycycline prophylaxis
Q fever	Vaccine (experimental) or tetracycline prophylaxis
Brucellosis	Doxycycline and rifampin prophylaxis
Tularemia	Vaccine (experimental) or tetracycline prophylaxis
Smallpox	Vaccine
Venezuelan equine encephalitis	Vaccine (experimental)
Viral hemorrhagic fevers	Vaccine (experimental)
Botulinum	Vaccine

TABLE 5-9

GENERAL TRIAGE CATEGORIES FOR BIOLOGICAL PATIENTS

Minimal	All ambulatory patients
Delayed	Moderate to severe symptoms
Immediate	Respiratory failure or decompensated shock
Expectant	Pulseless or persistent decompensated shock despite adequate IV fluids

As in all triage, it is essential to continually reassess and retriage patients as appropriate. Most biological patients will progress over time, much as natural disease does. Unlike chemical casualties, most biological casualties will take hours to worsen rather than minutes. This affords the EMS provider the opportunity to summon the required help to treat and transport the patients.

SUMMARY

This chapter reviewed the medical effects of biological weapons. The principles of field emergency care and management were highlighted. Recognition and identification of biological patients were emphasized. The role of self-protection and decontamination when caring for biological patients was also discussed.

FURTHER READING

Medical Management of Biological Casualties. U.S. Army Research Institute of Infectious Diseases, 2d Ed, Ft Detrick, MD, 1996

Emergency Response to Terrorism: Basic Concepts Student Manual. US Fire Administration, National Fire Academy. Emmitsburg, MD, 1997

FRANZ DR, et al: Clinical recognition and management of patients exposed to biological warfare agents. JAMA 1997; 278: 399-411

HOLLOWAY HC, et al: The threat of biological weapons. JAMA 1997; 278: 425-427 Christopher GW, et al: Biological warfare: A historical perspective. JAMA 1997; 278: 412-417

SPIERS EM: Chemical and Biological Weapons. St. Martin's Press, New York, 1984

ZAJTCHUK R, et al (eds): Medical Aspects of Chemical and Biological Warfare. Department of the Army, Office of the Surgeon General, Washington, DC, 1997

BORAK J, et al: Hazardous Materials Exposure. Prentice-Hall, Englewood cliffs, NJ, 1991

6

CARE OF NUCLEAR INJURIES

INTRODUCTION

The extensive United States effort to develop a nuclear bomb in the 1940s set the stage for utilization of the atom's awesome power. The wartime detonations over Nagasaki and Hiroshima, Japan and the accident at Chernobyl, USSR, demonstrate the potential for both wartime and peacetime casualty generation. Serious injury and death can also be associated with nuclear fuel or weapon transportation accidents and terrorist acts. The injuries produced by nuclear detonations and accidents can occur from several mechanisms and challenge the assessment and care skills of the EMS provider. To better respond to this challenge, let us look at the nuclear explosion, how it produces energy, and, ultimately, how it produces casualties.

THE NUCLEAR EXPLOSION

Conventional munitions gain their explosive power by breaking or changing the chemical bonds within the ordinance molecules. The result is kinetic energy, generally expressed as heat. (Heat is the measurement of molecule movement in a substance.) Nuclear energy is generated as the bonds inside the atom, and specifically the center of the atom (the nucleus) are broken and rearranged. Nuclear bonds are much stronger than chemical bonds; hence, they release much more energy when broken. Table 1-6 (chapter 1, Medical Aspects of WMD) outlines some of the destructive power of nuclear energy when harnessed as a bomb.

Nuclear Fusion/Fission

There are two types of nuclear reactions, fusion and fission. Fission breaks apart a large and unstable nucleus into multiple, smaller, and somewhat more stable nuclei. To create a reaction, forms (isotopes) of uranium and plutonium are pushed into high concentrations, inter-react, release energy and particles and form more stable atoms. This reaction is controlled to generate power and was used in the nuclear weapons of World War Two.

Fusion takes small atoms and fuses them into heavier ones. The reaction uses isotopes of hydrogen to form helium and other heavier elements. This process generates much more energy than fission but requires tremendous heat before a chain reaction can occur. The sun is an example of the fusion process. Science is not yet able to create a controlled fusion reaction because it is difficult to control the heat required to initiate and continue the reaction. For warfare, the necessary heat is generated by detonating a fission bomb within a concentration of fusion materials.

The Chain Reaction

In fission, an unstable nucleus divides (decays), forming more stable atoms and releasing heat and high-energy rays and particles. This occurs over time and is the radioactivity we associate with unstable isotopes. To create a chain reaction the concentration of radioactive material must be greatly enhanced. Then, when an isotope decays and releases high-energy particles, they collide with other unstable isotopes, causing them to decay and release more high-energy particles, and so on (Figure 6-1). If there is enough reactive material (a critical mass), the reaction rate grows dramatically and an explosion occurs. This process occurs in but a few thousandths of a second, creating great quantities of heat and electromagnetic energy that vaporize and blow the bomb apart. Only about 20% of the bomb's active nuclear material is responsible for the reaction and explosion.

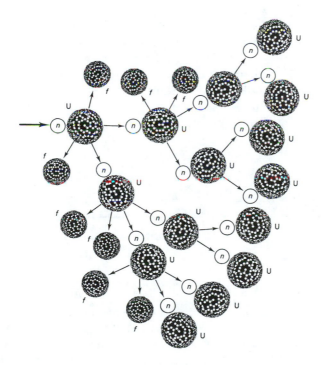

Figure 6-1 The chain reaction of the fission process.

As a chain reaction occurs, the heat energy and outflow of radiation become extreme. The great heat vaporizes the surrounding bomb casing and unspent nuclear fuel and creates the first flash of nuclear ignition. The reaction releases extremely concentrated X-ray, gamma, and neutron radiation that superheats the surrounding air. This forms the powerful second flash and fireball associated with a nuclear blast. The rapidly expanding, vaporized, and superheated material creates a shockwave and begins to rise from the ignition point (called ground zero). The superheated surrounding air rises rapidly and draws air, and possibly debris, in from underneath the explosion. This material too is vaporized and bombarded with radiation, becoming unstable (radioactive). It rises, cools, and condenses with the residual materials from the bomb (the characteristic mushroom cloud) forming small, radioactive particles that fall to earth as fallout. These events are responsible for the injury mechanisms associated with a nuclear detonation.

Fusion reactions create the same injury mechanisms as a fission detonation, however, they are generally much more powerful and also create a burst of electricity (called an electromagnetic pulse). Free electrons released from the reaction transmit an electrical surge outward. This current flow is extremely intense, and while it does not effect humans, it can have devastating effects on electrical equipment. Computers, medical diagnostic devices, communications equipment, and, in many cases, vehicles may be rendered inoperative. This may impact communications and your ability to arrange for transport and request supplies and assistance.

The energy expended by nuclear ignition differs greatly from a conventional explosion. The smallest of nuclear weapons (a tactical fission weapon weighing about 100 kg.) delivers the conventional explosive energy equivalent of five hundred tons (0.5 kiloton) of TNT. More modern fusion weapons deliver multimegatons (one million tons of TNT equivalent) of energy upon detonation. This energy is distributed among the blast wave, heat energy, and radiation (Figure 6-2). Fifty percent of the bomb's energy is in the blast wave (converted from initial thermal energy) while thirty-five percent is released as direct thermal energy. The remaining fifteen percent is released as initial radiation (5%) and radioactive debris (fallout, 10%). Some bombs are designed to distribute more initial radiation (approaching 30% of total output) and less physical destruction and fallout. These radiation enhanced or "dirty" bombs (Figure 6-3) are in the smaller range of nuclear arms and injure more personnel and fewer structures upon detonation.

NUCLEAR INJURY MECHANISMS

Nuclear detonation yields injury or death through three mechanisms. They are radiation, blast, and thermal burns.

Radiation

When an unstable (radioactive) atom breaks apart, it releases energy in the form of rays and particles traveling at high speeds (nuclear radiation). This nuclear or ionizing radiation differs from other types of radiation (light, heat, and sound) because it can change the structure of molecules it passes. These rays and particles damage the cells of the human body. The cells either die, repair themselves, or go on to produce damaged cells.

Nuclear Explosion Energy

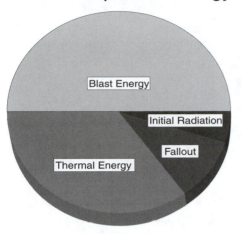

Figure 6-2 Bomb energy distribution of a typical nuclear bomb.

Nuclear Explosion Energy

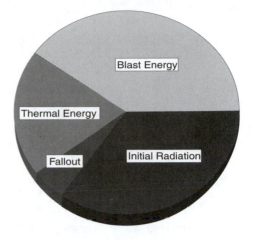

Figure 6-3 Bomb energy distribution of a radiation enhanced nuclear bomb.

We are constantly bombarded by ionizing radiation from natural sources (the stars, the sun, and the earth) with little if any ill effects. However, the concentration of radiation from a nuclear chain reaction or fallout is much more intense and life endangering. X-ray, gamma, neutron, beta, and alpha radiation are the most common radiations associated with fusion, fission, and fallout (Figure 6-4).

X-ray and Gamma Radiation

X-ray and gamma radiation are the same type of radiation though they are created by different processes. This powerful radiation is the most penetrating and occurs as unstable nuclei release energy and become more stable. The radiation is capable of traveling through one to two thousand meters of air, penetrating deeply into all but the densest of materials and damaging body cells in its path. X-ray and gamma radiation is generated in the reactor or bomb, and through the decay of radioactive particles, as in fallout. It is also given off when molecules are bombarded with high-speed electrons, as in the x-ray machine. Gamma radiation is the major external and, to a lesser extent, internal hazard associated with the nuclear detonation or reactor accident.

Neutron Radiation

Neutron radiation is released as the fission chain reaction occurs. It is a powerful and very damaging energy particle that penetrates several hundred meters of air and easily passes through the body. Since it occurs infrequently outside the nuclear chain reaction, its greatest threat to life occurs in close proximity to an active nuclear reactor or bomb ignition. For the sake of simplicity, neutron radiation, which does not penetrate as well as gamma radiation and X-rays, is considered along with this more penetrating radiation.

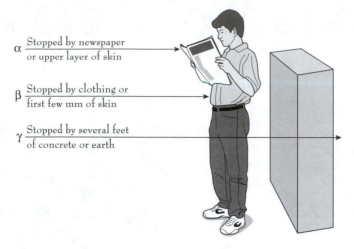

α — Stopped by newspaper or upper layer of skin

β — Stopped by clothing or first few mm of skin

γ — Stopped by several feet of concrete or earth

Figure 6-4 Relative penetrating power of nuclear radiation.

Beta Radiation

Beta radiation is a low-speed, low-energy particle that is easily stopped by six to ten feet of air, clothing, or the first few millimeters (or in some cases of high energy beta radiation, the first centimeter) of skin. It is a common byproduct of fallout decay and is a serious internal hazard from ingestion of contaminated food or inhalation of airborne, contaminated particles. While beta radiation is easily stopped by a few millimeters of soft tissue, it will cause significant ionization of those tissues.

Alpha Radiation

Alpha radiation is a very heavy and slow moving particle that travels only inches in air and is stopped by clothing or the outer layer of skin. It is a very serious internal contaminant because it causes a great amount of damage along its short course of travel. As with beta radiation, the greatest hazard of alpha radiation is inhalation or ingestion of the source (radioactive) material.

RADIATION EXPOSURE

There are two types of radiation exposure associated with the nuclear explosion. They are the primary exposure associated with the intense nuclear reaction and fallout.

Primary Radiation Exposure

Serious primary radiation injury during and shortly after a nuclear detonation is limited. The rising fireball draws the radioactive materials upward and away from the ground very quickly, with exposure occurring for only the first minute immediately after detonation. Neutron and gamma radiation also travel only one to two thousand meters through air so exposure is limited to the blast proximity. Hence, for most nuclear weapons, the mortality caused by primary radiation is overshadowed by blast and thermal injuries. The only exception is the small, radiation-enhanced tactical weapon, where radiation doses may be sufficient to kill while the blast strength and thermal injury may not.

When exposure to radioactive energy occurs due to a nondetonation experience, such as a reactor or transportation accident, gamma radiation is the most serious hazard. While these exposures are not as intense as the radiation exposure associated with an uncontrolled chain reaction, they can result in severe and life-threatening injury to persons near the source of radiation. Here the radioactive source strength, the exposure duration, any shielding, and the distance from the source directly effect the potential for injury and death.

Fallout

The second form of radiation exposure is fallout. Fallout is radioactive dust and particles that may present life-threatening hazards not only near the blast epicenter but some distance away. As the superheated products of nuclear detonation and surrounding debris are drawn up and into the atmosphere, they are bombarded with nuclear reaction byproducts, energized, and then distributed by winds aloft (and not always in the same direction as surface winds) (Figure 6-5). If the nuclear detonation occurs at or close to the ground, the updraft of debris is increased, as is the amount of fallout.

The radioactive material may be scattered anywhere from a few miles surrounding ground zero to around the world. The most immediately dangerous radiation falls shortly

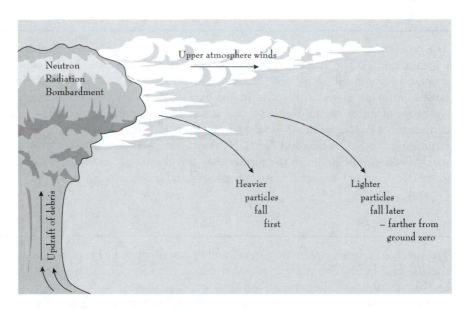

Figure 6-5 Process of nuclear fallout creation and deposition.

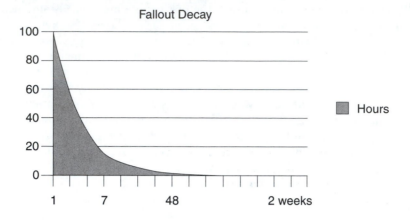

Figure 6-6 Fallout strength decay.

after and (within forty-eight hours) in close proximity to the blast, in the form of larger, heavier particles. This fallout is the most hazardous because it is concentrated over a relatively small geographic area. It is an intense ionizing radiation source since it has not had much time to decay (Figure 6-6).

A similar condition to fallout occurring during a reactor accident is the release of radioactive particles or gasses. While the area of coverage and radiation intensity are not as great as with a bomb, the health risk is still serious.

BLAST

The rapid heating of air surrounding the nuclear ignition creates an explosively expanding gas cloud. As the cloud's outward movement reaches the speed of sound, it creates a shockwave and a following blast of wind. The shockwave and blast wind produce the same injuries associated with conventional explosives, though the intensity close to and the range of injury outward from ground zero are much, much greater. The blast winds can reach over 160 miles-per-hour and may displace personnel and topple structures, resulting in further trauma and death. However, like radiation, the shockwave and blast wind effects rapidly diminish the further they travel from ground zero. Blast is discussed in greater detail in Chapter 3, Care of Explosive and Incendiary Injuries.

THERMAL BURNS

The mechanism resulting in most injury and death associated with nuclear detonation is the thermal burn. The nuclear reaction releases tremendous thermal energy which, unlike radiation and blast energy, travels unimpeded through air to its target. There the energy is absorbed by the contact surface, creating burns or igniting combustibles. While the heating is of very short duration, it is extremely intense. Anything in close proximity to the detonation is incinerated. A ten megaton bomb will result in fifty percent mortality due to burns fourteen kilometers (ten miles) from ground zero.

While thermal injury is the most prevalent injury from nuclear weapons, it is the easiest injury to shield against. Any opaque object between the fireball and victim captures the energy. White or light colored clothing reflects much of the heat energy. The burn involves only the surface facing the detonation, but heat energy may ignite clothing or building materials, resulting in a flame burn.

Further out from the blast epicenter, thermal burns caused by the short duration flash appear very serious. However, they may involve only the epidermis and upper layers of dermis because of the short duration heat exposure and the skin's resistance to thermal injury. The prognosis for complete healing is very good, even with limited care, unless the burn is extensive or complicated by radiation exposure or trauma. Thermal burns caused by secondary mechanisms, such as clothing ignition, carry the same degree of seriousness as normal first, second, and third degree thermal burns. Burns are discussed in greater detail in Chapter 3, Care of Explosive and Incendiary Injuries.

One event sometimes associated with nuclear ignition, especially when the detonation area contains substantial combustibles, is a firestorm. The blast and extreme heat ignite flammable materials while the ensuing fire is fanned by air drawn into the rising mushroom cloud. The result is a region of intense heat and fire. Burns associated with such an event are extremely deadly.

Eye burn injuries may be associated with the brilliant light flash of nuclear detonation. The intense light may cause momentary blindness as the flash stuns the retina. As with a flash bulb in a dark room, the patient is blinded for a few seconds or minutes, or possibly for as long as thirty minutes when the flash occurs during the night. These effects completely disappear with time, though they can severely impair the patient's ability to function and care for himself/herself. If the patient looks directly at the detonation and focuses on the flash, the intense light may physically burn and permanently damage the retina. The injury destroys light sensitivity where the image focuses, but the patient retains peripheral vision over the remainder of the retina.

Concentric Circles of Injury and Destruction

The explosive energy of a nuclear detonation distributes outward from ground zero. As energy travels away from the blast center, it quickly dissipates. There is an inner most circle of complete destruction with flattened and burned buildings and foliage, and no personnel found alive. The next concentric circle contains much destruction to all but the stoutest of structures. Most victims suffer mortal injuries from radiation, the blast wave, and burns. Some victims may survive if they are shielded from the heat by objects between them and the blast, though many die from collapsing structures. The next circle has greater survival, with patients exposed to the flash suffering severe burns. The shockwave and radiation may induce serious injury, but thermal burns are the greatest cause of death. As the reaction energy moves further from ground zero, the primary radiation exposure drops off rapidly and pressure injuries diminish quickly. Burns remain the major cause of injury or death in these more distant circles. The more powerful the bomb, the larger the respective circles of destruction, injury, and death (Figure 6-7).

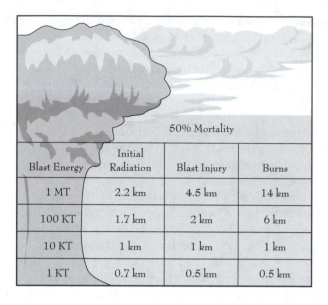

Blast Energy	Initial Radiation	Blast Injury	Burns
1 MT	2.2 km	4.5 km	14 km
100 KT	1.7 km	2 km	6 km
10 KT	1 km	1 km	1 km
1 KT	0.7 km	0.5 km	0.5 km

50% Mortality

Figure 6-7 Rings of nuclear destruction.

RADIATION EXPOSURE INJURY

Radiation exposure results in injury through different mechanisms than either thermal burns or injuries produced by the pressure of the blast. These injuries also manifest in ways different from conventional wounds.

Ionizing radiation travels through body tissue and may alter some cell structures. Most commonly, radiation damages the DNA or causes chemical changes which damage the DNA. Since DNA is a cell's blueprint for reproduction, cells that reproduce quickly manifest effects soonest and have the least time to effect DNA repairs and suffer most from radiation exposure. The cells, in descending order of sensitivity, are those of the bone marrow, blood, bowel, skin, and nervous and cardiovascular systems.

Bone Marrow and Blood Cells

Moderate doses of gamma and neutron radiation penetrate the body and damage red bone marrow and blood cells. The marrow generates blood cells that carry oxygen and those that help with immunity and clotting. A reduction in the blood's oxygen carrying capacity results in slight nausea, fatigue, and a general ill feeling (malaise). Later on, reduced platelet production induces clotting disorders and, possibly, uncontrollable hemorrhage. White blood cell destruction reduces the body's ability to rid itself of infection. The early signs and symptoms of bone marrow and blood cell injury usually take anywhere from four to thirty-six hours to become evident.

The radiation dosage necessary to damage the bone marrow and blood cells is generally survivable if not complicated by other injuries. However, when this early radiation syndrome is present, it is very important to reduce the patient's exposure to infection.

Any infection attacking the body when the white blood cell production is reduced may be severe and fatal.

Bowel

As the acute dosage increases, radiation penetrating the body begins to damage cells reproducing the bowel lining. This causes nausea, loss of appetite (anorexia), possible vomiting, diarrhea, fluid loss, and malaise. In later stages, dehydration and malnutrition, and bowel hemorrhage and perforation may occur. The early evidence of this syndrome appears a couple of hours after exposure and before those associated with bone marrow and blood cell damage. This syndrome may also result from the ingestion of food contaminated with emitters of alpha and beta particles, i.e., fallout. Internal contamination will take longer to produce signs and symptoms. Bowel damage and the resulting signs and symptoms usually suggest a lethal dose of primary radiation. However, with extensive supportive care, and if the radiation is not compounded by other injury, these patients can survive.

Skin

The upper layers of the dermis rapidly produce the dying skin cells of the body's surface. This rapid cell production makes the skin sensitive to ionizing radiation. The acute dosages creating gastrointestinal signs and symptoms often affect the skin. Cell damage causes a generalized skin reddening called erythema. While this injury does not significantly threaten the patient's life, it may reflect exposure to significant doses of beta, gamma and neutron radiation. Nonuniform erythema may suggest partial shielding from the radiation. However, a weapon's thermal flash may also redden or burn the skin and confound this sign's value for assessment.

Fallout may cover unprotected skin and, with time, subject it to alpha and beta radiation. The skin may redden as with sunburn. If exposure persists and the area is subjected to extremely high radiation dosages, more serious burns may occur.

Nervous and Cardiovascular Systems

With more acute radiation exposure, blood vessel and nerve cells are affected. The result is a rapid onset of incapacitation, cardiovascular collapse, confusion, and with very extreme doses, a burning or "on fire" sensation throughout the body. Dosages sufficient to cause nervous and vascular damage, and the associated signs and symptoms, are generally very severe and do not permit survival even with intensive, resource consuming efforts. This is especially true if the patient has sustained any thermal burn or blast injury.

Evaluating Exposure

As the radiation dosage increases, the signs and symptoms of exposure appear earlier and become more severe. The first signs of serious exposure are slight nausea and fatigue occurring within four to twenty-four hours after exposure. As the radiation dose moves into the lethal range, nausea severity increases and is accompanied by anorexia (lack of appetite), vomiting, diarrhea, and malaise. Erythema of the skin may be present and fatigue becomes more intense. These signs appear within two to six hours. With increasingly fatal doses, the patient displays all the signs of radiation exposure almost immediately, and later evidences confusion, watery diarrhea, and physical collapse.

With all the syndromes of radiation exposure, from the least to most serious, the patient will display initial illness signs and symptoms, may seem to get better, then gets worse. This occurs because the body attempts to repair itself after the initial damage. However, once the damaged cells fail to reproduce or produce damaged cells, a period of frank illness sets in. These phases of radiation sickness each span several days or weeks for the lesser doses and hours for extremely lethal radiation exposures. It should also be noted that there is a varied individual sensitivity to radiation exposure.

Cancer

Cancer is a flawed cell reproduction that becomes evident many years after serious radiation exposure and only in a small portion of those exposed. Since it is impossible to determine who this problem will affect and there is no care either to prevent or limit its development, you will not address this radiation exposure consequence.

NUCLEAR CASUALTY ASSESSMENT

Both the nuclear detonation and accident drastically change your role as an emergency care provider. Your major responsibilities will probably involve triage, evacuation or sheltering, search and rescue, radioactive monitoring, decontamination, and limited patient care. Let us examine the various nuclear scenarios and your respective scene size-up and initial responsibilities. These scenarios include the detonation (strategic, terrorist, and tactical) and the accident (reactor or fuel generation or transportation) .

NUCLEAR DETONATION

Detonation is most likely to be a strategic weapon explosion as part of a major offensive action, a single terrorist event, or a tactical event on the battlefield. Each type of explosion is very different in the magnitude of energy release, the effect it has on casualties and the care provision system, and on your responsibilities as a EMS provider.

Strategic Detonation

Strategic nuclear detonations will involve large urban or military locations and deliver multi-megatons of explosive energy. There will probably be numerous detonations, and the ability to obtain additional medical and evacuation support will be severely limited. Because the weapon is likely a fusion bomb with a significant electrical surge, available radio communications will be compromised, as will be most vehicle operation. You will probably be brought into the area as part of a mass effort to provide search and rescue, triage, evacuation, radiological monitoring, decontamination, and some limited care.

Your initial assignment at a strategic nuclear detonation will be primarily search and rescue, followed by staging in anticipation of evacuation. Size-up the scene to determine the degree of radiation hazard, both on the ground and from fallout. Be sure you and your team are protected from the effects of any radioactive fallout (don personal protective equipment and personal dosimeters). Take a quick inventory of care supplies, methods of transportation, and personnel to assist with patient movement. Determine what additional resources, if any, might be available. Find a suitable location for staging patients in anticipation of evacuation. Ideally this area will not be downwind from ground zero. This will minimize fallout accumulation. If you anticipate a delay between staging and transportation and there is a serious risk of fallout, select a large structure with a protected interior. The greater the distance between casualties and the accumulating radioactive fallout, the lower the risk from continuing exposure. The center of the basement of a large, stable, multifloor structure is best.

Search and rescue starts at the outer perimeter of injury and destruction and works inward, clearing routes of travel along the way. Egress to casualties may be the greatest obstacle to the response effort as trees, collapsed buildings, disabled vehicles, and other debris litter the disaster scene. As you find casualties, extricate them from debris and arrange for assisted movement to the staging area (if they are nonambulatory). As you move closer to ground zero, the severity and incidence of burn injuries increases and starts to mix with pressure injuries to the ears, lungs and bowel. Closer to ground zero, the burn and pressure injuries become critical and join with moderate, then serious radiation exposure.

If medical personnel are in short supply, staff the staging area to provide triage and limited supportive care. As more EMS personnel become available, direct them to work with the search and rescue teams. They will provide triage and immediate life-saving care only. Because of the fallout hazard, all immediate, minimal, delayed, and ambulatory expectant casualties are sent to the staging area, then evacuated to fallout-secure locations.

Since the ability to obtain outside help for one of many strategic detonation areas is limited, some other resources will be critical to patient survival. The devastation caused by the blast will destroy most sources of potable water, food, power, clothing, heat, and shelter. During your search and rescue activities and whenever outside the fallout zone, look for resources that may help meet these needs as the disaster progresses. Protect food and water sources from contamination. Assure adequate shelter from the environment and begin to acquire medical supplies (like clean fabric, makeshift splints, etc.) Locate lighting and power sources such as flashlights and operating vehicles.

Also assure proper sanitary facilities. In the disaster environment, infection quickly becomes a major concern due to poor sanitation and the decreased infection fighting capability of casualties. Isolate the water supply and sanitation. Be sure food is well-cooked, eating utensils are clean, and water is boiled if necessary. Isolate the injured from the dead and from any other source of infection.

Tactical Detonation

Tactical nuclear detonation occurs on the battlefield with the purpose of destroying the enemy's will and ability to fight. The tactical nuclear weapon is of limited yield and possibly radiation enhanced. For the most part, use of tactical nuclear weapons is restricted to battles and wars and will not be directly addressed here. The effect of a tactical detonation will likely fall between that of a terrorist (small) and strategic (large) detonation.

Terrorist Detonation

Terrorist nuclear detonation will probably be limited to one small (one to multi-kiloton) detonation in a highly populated area. It is likely that national resources will rapidly be brought to the scene and massive evacuation and extensive care will be possible during the days thereafter. However, during the first few hours of the disaster, resources are severely limited and the damage to structures and personnel is great. You will assist with search and rescue, monitor radiation levels, evacuate casualties, or, at a remote location, provide supportive care. Your actions will probably be directed by a civilian incident command system.

After a terrorist nuclear detonation, your role may be similar to that associated with the strategic detonation. However, the available resources are much greater and the structural damage and number of casualties much reduced. Evacuation and shelter are given high priority due to the radioactive fallout hazard. Intensive scene and hospital care is offered to all patients who need it, though immediate category patients will receive it first. The incident command system will designate medical sectors such as extrication (search and rescue), triage, treatment, and transport. Because of the incident size, there may be several sectors established geographically for each designation.

NUCLEAR ACCIDENTS

Nuclear accidents are usually isolated incidents effecting only those personnel in close proximity to the reactor or leak. On rare occasions, the accident may be a major incident contaminating many square miles and endangering hundreds of thousands of people. The nuclear accident's ability to cause property damage or personnel injury is much less than that of even the smallest nuclear weapon. The vast majority of accidents present serious radiation exposures to few personnel and very limited radiation exposure to the population. Nuclear accidents are most likely reactor or fuel processing, or transportation accidents. A terrorist act of sabotage on a nuclear power plant or transport asset may result in effects similar to a nuclear accident. Conventional explosives attached to a radiation source will, when detonated, also cause similar radiation effcets. The principles outlined in this section apply to all these possibilities.

Reactor or Fuel Processing Accident

Reactor accidents can be serious because there is a relatively large quantity of nuclear material present and there is also a chain reaction taking place. While a nuclear explosion is not possible, intense heat or pressure may damage the reactor and its containment vessel. The result may be a release of radioactive steam or vapor and the danger of contamination. There may also be internal accidents involving the handling of radioactive materials. These accidents subject a very small number of personnel to radiation danger, though their injuries may be severe.

Fuel processing accidents occur during nuclear fuel enrichment for use in power or research reactors or in weapons. It is unlikely that a critical mass is present and that an explosion will occur. However, the reaction may become uncontrolled, creating great heat and releasing radioactive steam, smoke and vapor into the atmosphere, or injuring plant personnel. Personnel may also be seriously or mortally injured if the shielding is compromised.

Expect reactor or plant personnel, under the direction of the health physicists, to provide any fire fighting, radiation containment, and clean-up services. Your role as an EMS provider will likely be to evacuate or shelter civilians, monitor radioactivity, or provide decontamination services. These services are guided by reactor or plant personnel.

Transportation Accidents

Transportation accidents can occur whenever radioactive materials are moved. The material can be intended for medical treatment or diagnosis, reactor fuels, industrial testing agents, radioactive waste, or weapon production. Radioactive material is only shipped in very small quantities or in crash-proof containers. Leaks or spills only effect a small and immediate area unless combustion from other agents, aerosolizes the material.

An exception occurs when nuclear weapons are damaged through air travel and high-velocity crashes. While nuclear weapons are safeguarded against ignition, the conventional explosives used to induce the nuclear detonation may explode on impact. Weapon-grade nuclear material is then scattered around the crash site and poses a hazard within the debris perimeter. Any further combustion, as with jet fuel, may introduce the radiation into the atmosphere.

In the transportation accident, you may be called to monitor radioactivity or to assist with evacuation and, rarely, decontamination. Since casualties are unlikely, and radiation exposure is limited, you will probably not provide much medical care. The exception might be a military aircraft crash into a populated area where you may render care for trauma and burn injuries not associated with radiation exposure.

ASSESSMENT

When assessing nuclear detonation casualties, remember that this is a disaster, and assessment and triage must occur quickly. Visually sweep each patient for any signs of serious injury, most likely burns, or blunt trauma. Check quickly for signs and symptoms of pressure injuries, especially any lung injury, difficulty breathing, or small stroke-like symptoms (air emboli). Note the distance from the explosion center and any early complaints of radiation exposure such as nausea or fatigue.

During a mass casualty incident, such as a detonation or serious accident, document your patient assessment and care well. Be sure you record the patient's initial location and describe each serious injury and complaint. Identify the time after exposure that the patient complains of any radiation related signs and symptoms. This information will help to determine the radiation dosage and the ultimate triage category assigned the patient.

TRIAGE

Triage is a difficult responsibility for anyone involved with a nuclear event, especially a detonation. The signs and symptoms of serious radiation exposure may not occur for several hours and are not suggestive of imminent death. Sensitivity to radiation exposure varies greatly from individual to individual, and sub lethal radiation exposure, when combined with other serious injuries, greatly increases mortality. With these considerations in mind, let us look at triage approaches in evaluating nuclear detonation and nuclear accident casualties.

Nuclear Explosion Triage

Before employing a triage system at a nuclear explosion, carefully evaluate the resources you have at hand or that will become available. When resources (medical personnel, supplies, and transportation) are adequate or will arrive soon, limit the expectant category to those who will die despite intensive care. In the strategic or tactical weapon deployment, you may be forced to triage patients as expectant who could otherwise survive with only moderate care. To act differently reduces the chance of survival for others who need less extensive care.

It is best to begin the triage process from the outer ring of destruction. Here the primary mechanism of injury is the burns. While burns may look severe and, in some cases, charred, the quick delivery of the blast's thermal energy reduces the burn depth. Check for the absence of pain, indicating full thickness burns, and use the rule of nines to approximate burn surface area. Each adult body region (each arm, the head, the anterior chest, the posterior chest, the anterior abdomen, the posterior abdomen, each anterior leg, and each posterior leg) is approximately 9% of the total surface area. See chapter 3, Care of Explosive amd Incendiary Injuries for details on "Rule of 9s" calculations.

Categorize any 70% (50% in the elderly or chronically ill) or greater full thickness burn as expectant. Classify any burns greater than 20% full thickness as delayed. Any serious burn involving a joint area or circumferentially covering a limb or the trunk is increased in severity by one position, as are those affecting the very young, old or anyone with a pre-existing or concurrent disease or serious injury. If the burn is complicated by any signs of respiratory burn injury, also move the patient's triage category one closer to immediate.

As you move closer to ground zero, the depth and severity of burns increase and this mechanism of injury is joined by pressure injuries. Designate casualties with serious signs of lung injuries as expectant, moderate or minor lung injury signs as immediate, bowel injury signs as delayed, and ear injury signs as minimal. This concentric destruction and injury ring may also produce blunt trauma from blast wind projectiles, patient displacement, or collapsing structures. Move any serious mixed injuries (any two or more of burn, pressure, or blunt trauma) one triage category toward expectant.

The next closest ring of destruction introduces radiation injuries along with increasingly severe burn, pressure, and blunt trauma injuries. Here burns, pressure injuries, and radiation each account for a mortality greater than 50%. It is unlikely that many casualties will be found alive, and those that are are likely to die regardless of the care you provide. Place only those casualties with limited injuries and no early signs of radiation exposure in the immediate category. All others are expectant.

Sorting casualties for radiation exposure is difficult because the signs are delayed and are often intermingled with other, more apparent injuries. Signs suggestive of moderate radiation exposure include mild to moderate nausea, vomiting, possible diarrhea, and fever. In severe radiation exposure the patient will display severe nausea, vomiting, and mild to severe diarrhea and fever. The severely irradiated patient may also display erythema, hypotension, and CNS dysfunction. Remember, as the primary radiation dose increases, the signs become more severe and appear sooner. During your early triage (the first few hours), patients presenting with signs and symptoms of radiation injury are most likely to have the most serious exposure.

Triaging casualties into the expectant category is a difficult task in any nuclear detonation. Patients who receive lethal radiation doses appear sick but certainly not mortally injured. You must simply comfort them without providing extensive care because those with a chance of survival need your services and supplies. You may also note that many radiation casualties seem to improve with time. Due to the nature of radiation injury, this improvement is transient, will be followed by more serious signs and symptoms, and does not indicate that the patient will survive.

Nuclear Accident Triage

The nuclear accident is a much easier situation to triage. The emergency medical service system is intact and supplies, personnel, and transportation are or will be available in adequate quantities. The accident is also likely to produce fewer, less serious radiation exposures and few, if any, thermal burns or pressure injuries. In the nuclear accident, it is unlikely that you will employ disaster triage.

The major injuries associated with a radiation accident will be radiation exposure and, possibly, radiation burns. Upon arrival at the scene, locate the health physics staff and function under their direction. In their absence, place yourself at a distance from the site with some large mass of steel, concrete or earth between you and the radiation source. Identify the location and number of victims, and, if possible, the level of radiation. If there is a danger of fallout or radioactive smoke, steam or other contamination, don protective equipment. Attempt a patient rescue if the expected total rescuer exposure will be 25 rem or less. Have the rescuers don dosimeters and be sure they move quickly toward the patient and then away from the source. Decontaminate the patient as necessary, then transport.

Radiation exposure injuries, most commonly skin burns, do not occur for hours unless the exposure is from extremely strong gamma radiation or is a result of prolonged surface contamination with alpha and beta emitting particles. Simply provide decontamination as needed and care for the associated burns as you would for thermal burns.

NUCLEAR INJURY CARE

The scene size-up and assessment determines whether radiation exposure is due to a nuclear detonation, fallout at some distance from the conflagration, or an isolated noncritical mass incident. Each of these mechanisms of injury and exposure calls for you to perform different activities as an EMS provider. These activities are common to the scenarios mentioned earlier and include search and rescue, transportation and sheltering, decontamination, and supportive medical care.

SEARCH AND RESCUE

After donning personal protective equipment and dosimeters, the next step is to locate casualties. Search and rescue is an essential part of the nuclear detonation response, as patients may be trapped or isolated by debris. In most nuclear detonations, as you get closer to the area of extreme destruction, travel becomes more difficult. Once a patient is found, there may be difficulties in removing them from the scene and to the staging area.

Usually the responsibility for search and rescue will be left to nonmedical personnel. The EMS provider's knowledge and skills are needed at the staging area for triage and limited on-scene care, or at a remote location for decontamination and supportive care.

When removing casualties from a radiation accident, reduce rescuer exposure by minimizing exposure time, maintaining the greatest distance possible from the radioactive source, and using natural and artificial shielding. Have rescuers move to the patient and bring him/her out of the area as quickly as possible. Radioactive exposure is a cumulative danger so shorter exposures are less damaging. Transport patients to a distant location. Radiation strength falls off very quickly with increasing distance from the source. Also use any natural shielding such as earthen berms, ditches or heavy building walls between you and the source to reduce exposure. Lastly, since cancer is a significant but very delayed effect of radiation exposure, utilize older rescuers to perform actions that will garner the greatest radiation doses. Their shorter remaining life span reduces the chance of cancer developing. If it does develop, it will likely occur at a later age.

EVACUATION AND SHELTERING

Evacuation removes casualties from the danger associated with radioactive fallout. You will generally place casualties perpendicular to the wind direction. This moves them quickly to a safe zone. However, wind direction changes frequently, so watch for wind shifts and continue moving the casualties to safety. Radiologic monitoring will help guide evacuation and help you seek shelter from exposure while waiting for transportation,.

If medical support personnel are in adequate supply, you may ride with casualties during evacuation. During this time, care for the patients triaged to immediate, delayed, and minimal categories and provide comfort (psychological support and empathy) to the expectant. You will most likely treat thermal burns, pressure injuries, and blunt trauma.

If transportation is not possible, shelter personnel from fallout and radioactive contamination. Sheltering is best accomplished by placing as much distance and substance between you and the accumulating radioactive material. Two inches of steel, six of concrete, eight of earth, and twenty-two of wood, will each reduce radiation gamma radiation exposure by fifty percent. If fallout is, or you expect it to become, a significant exposure threat, locate or construct a shelter.

EMERGENCY CARE

Emergency medical care at the nuclear incident, be it detonation or accident, is limited. Due to the nature of a detonation, a restrictive triage must be employed to salvage the greatest number of casualties. Conversely, the radiation accident, even with high personal exposures, does not produce wounds that need immediate care. The only injuries requiring your attention are conventional burns and blunt or pressure injuries. There are helpful guidelines regarding the typical injuries associated with a nuclear incident.

Conventional (Thermal) Burn Care

Thermal burns associated with the tremendous heat of a nuclear detonation can be severe. Attend to them as you would any burn while taking special care to reduce potential infection. Since radiation exposure suppresses the immune system, the body will be less able to combat the serious infections often associated with full thickness burns.

Since burns induced by nuclear explosion heat cover a large portion of the body's surface, care for them by covering the area with clean dressings. While sterile burn sheets are ideal, in an area of mass destruction, freshly laundered bedsheets are a reasonable substitute. If adjacent skin surfaces, such as the hands or feet, are seriously burned, place non-adherent dressings between the digits. This keeps the injury surfaces from adhering to each other. If the body was well shielded and burns only affect small surfaces, cover them with smaller sterile dressings.

Serious burns can quickly cause dehydration. Third degree burns break down the skin and its function as a container for the human body. Fluid seeps through the wound and evaporates. The result is rapid dehydration and possible hypothermia. First and second degree burns also increase the likelihood of hypothermia because they dilate the surface blood vessels, permitting a rapid loss of heat to the environment. Maintain the body temperature of any patient with extensive first, second, and third degree burns.

Consider fluid administration if IV solutions are in adequate supply. Administer a bolus of 1,000 milliliters of normal saline (pediatrics 20 ml/kg) in the first hour after a third degree burn affecting more than 20% of the body surface area. Administer additional fluid as for conventionally caused burns. Pain medication may also be helpful for the serious or extensive burn patient. Administer morphine sulfate in 2 mg increments until pain relief, a reduced level of consciousness, or a total of 10 mg has been administered. Repeat the dosing as needed for pain. In general, antibiotics are contraindicated in the initial phase of burn care.

Injuries to the eyes caused by the detonation blast will require little specific care. The flash blindness lasts only a few minutes during daylight and as long as thirty minutes at night. Assure patients that their eyesight will return shortly and have a buddy remain with them until it does. With retinal burns, the blindness is more permanent, though patients will have peripheral vision and be able to move about and provide basic care for themselves after a short period of adjustment. No emergency medical care is needed for either condition. Chapter 3, Care of Explosive and Incendiary Injuries, provides additional details on aspects of burn care.

Blunt Trauma Care

Trauma associated with a nuclear detonation will be blunt in nature and anywhere from mild to extremely serious. Injuries occur from debris placed in motion by the blast wind, casualties thrown by the wind, and structural collapse. Fractured limbs, possible spinal injury, head and torso blunt trauma, and penetrating trauma caused by flying glass and other sharp debris are common. Care for these wounds in accordance with standard emergency care principles.

Fallout danger may require rapid transportation of patients before you can completely stabilize their wounds. Secure the arms to the torso, tie the legs together, and move casualties to the stretcher along the long axis of the body. Protect the head as you move the patient. Care for specific injuries will likely occur after triage and evacuation.

Pressure Trauma Care

Pressure injuries of greatest concern are those affecting the lungs. The damage and tearing of the alveoli causes swelling, fluid accumulation, and, possibly, pulmonary emboli.

Progressive swelling and fluid accumulation make breathing more labored and less efficient with time. Oxygen has a more difficult time getting into the blood stream and the patient becomes hypoxic. If any lung pressure injury signs are present, administer 100% oxygen. Use positive pressure ventilation only when necessary and then only to obtain moderate chest rise and air movement. Lung tissue damage may allow air to directly enter the blood stream and seriously threaten life. If you suspect pulmonary emboli, place the patient in a head-down position on his/her left side. This will slow the movement of air bubbles into the systemic circulation. Monitor respirations and watch for developing dyspnea and possible tension pneumothorax. If you suspect tension pneumothorax, consider pleural decompression.

Ear and bowel injury caused by the blast pressure wave require only supportive care. Bowel injury presents with abdominal pain and needs no immediate field treatment other than making the patient as comfortable as possible. If there is ear pain and/or hearing loss, keep the ear (auditory) canal clean, make the patient as comfortable as is possible, and suspect possible lung damage. Remember, patients with diminished hearing will need psychological support and reassurance. Chapter 3, Care of Explosive and Incendiary Injuries, provides additional details on aspects of blast injury and pressure trauma care.

Radiation Exposure Considerations

The effects of severe radiation exposure, if they are indeed survivable, present after a few hours. Damage is diffuse throughout the body and the only helpful care is antibiotic therapy and rehydration. Unless you are with the patient for a prolonged period of time and resources are adequate to care for large numbers of patients, little field care can be offered for the radiation-exposed patient.

When radiation exposure is combined with other trauma, direct special attention to keeping wounds clean and reducing the chances of infection. Radiation exposure will limit the body's ability to fight off infection and the introduction of infectious agents through any wound will seriously threaten the patient's life. Consider irrigating any wound with potential contamination, apply sterile dressings, and later, in care, use antibiotic therapy under the supervision of a physician.

In areas of increased exposure to radiation due to detonation fallout, you may be called to help with oral administration of sodium iodine to the population. A detonation by product, radioactive iodine, enters the food chain and becomes concentrated in the thyroid. Thyroid cell damage caused by this concentration and radioactive decay may lead to an increased incidence of cancer. Administration of nonradioactive iodine saturates the organ, reduces any radiation concentration, and reduces the risk of thyroid cancer. Unit (single) dose tablets of sodium iodine are taken orally, once per day. The risk from radioactive iodine lasts for a few weeks, during which time you may be asked to distribute or administer the tablets.

Occasionally, you may treat a patient with a localized and severe radiation exposure. This is likely to occur during the handling of gamma-emitting radioactive material. Here the damage is limited to a small portion of the body and the injury area is well defined. The patient will suffer severe burns, manifest an intense local burning sensation and develop weeping wounds within a few hours. These wounds are best covered with sterile dressings and attended by a physician trained in radiation injury care.

SUMMARY

Nuclear detonation energy is released as light and thermal energy, a shock wave and blast of wind, and direct radiation, then fallout. Potential injuries include the following: light damage to the eye, and burns to the skin, blast (pressure) injury, injury associated with being hit by propelled objects being thrown by the blast of wind, radiation from bomb ignition and from falling radioactive particles. These injury mechanisms often combine during nuclear detonation, presenting an assessment and care challenge. Understanding the injury process associated with nuclear detonation aids in anticipating, assessing, triaging, and caring for casualties.

Your role at a nuclear disaster or accident is very different from that of normal emergency care. In a disaster, triage shifts to placing many casualties into the expectant category due to limited resources and the massive damage caused by the nuclear detonation. Most casualties are burned, though some may suffer pressure or blunt trauma. A few may have serious radiation exposure, show few signs, yet may die without intensive supportive care. Your role at the disaster is to provide search and rescue, triage, radioactivity monitoring, evacuation, decontamination, and limited emergency care.

In an accident, assessment and care are more conventional and are probably guided by incident command system or health physics personnel. Your role is to monitor radiation levels, and support evacuation and decontamination. Injuries and radiation exposure are limited, as is the extent of emergency care you provide.

FOR FURTHER READING

Textbook of Military Medicine (Part 1, Volume 2) Medical Consequences of Nuclear Warfare. Office of the Surgeon General, Washington, D.C. 1990

MEYER, E.: Chemistry of Hazardous Materials, 2nd Edition. Prentice-Hall, Englewood Cliffs, NJ. 1989.

Manual of Protective Action Guidelines and Protective Action for Nuclear Incidents: Environmental Protection Agency, Washington, D.C. 1992 (EPA-400-R-92-001)

CASARETT, A.: Radiation Biology: Prentice-Hall, Englewood Cliffs, NJ 1968

GRACE, C.: Nuclear Weapons: Principles, Effects and Survivability, Brassey's Limited, London, UK. 1995

CHRISTEN, H., MANISCALCO, P.: The EMS Incident Management System: EMS Operations for Mass Casualty and High Impact Incidents. Prentice-Hall, Upper Saddle River, NJ 1998.

AUF DER HEIDE, E.: Disaster Response: Principles of Preparation and Coordination. C. V. Mosby Company, St. Louis, MO. 1989

MEYER E: Chemistry of Hazardous Materials, 3rd ed. Prentice-Hall, Upper Saddle River, NJ 1998

7

PERSONAL PROTECTION AND PATIENT DECONTAMINATION

PROTECTION FROM NBC AGENTS

Overview

Personal protection is a critical element in providing safe and effective care to patients exposed to nuclear, biological or chemical (NBC) agents. Only through personal protection you prevent illness or injury to yourself as you care for these types of patients. Personal protection will involves wearing specialized equipment and clothes. This ensemble is collectively called personal protective equipment (PPE) and may include a mask, overgarment, gloves and boots. It is important that all EMS providers be thoroughly familiar with the PPE they will be expected to don and wear during a WMD operation. This chapter will introduce the concepts needed by EMS providers to operate safely in an NBC contaminated environment, but is not intended as a thorough or complete reference. Readers desiring more information are encouraged to review one of the many fine textbooks on hazardous materials in the fire, rescue and EMS literature.

Zones

When dealing with a hazardous material such as an NBC agent, the incident commander will establish areas or zones based on the estimate of contamination in the area. In general terms, the zones can be envisioned as concentric circles with the hot or most contaminated zone in the center (Figure 7-1), like a bull's-eye target. The next ring is the warm zone, an area of potential contamination, but much less hazardous than the hot zone. The outermost ring is the cold zone, which represents the areas unaffected by the contaminant. Factors affecting the size and shape of the zones include the toxicity and persistence of the agent, wind conditions, and sunlight.

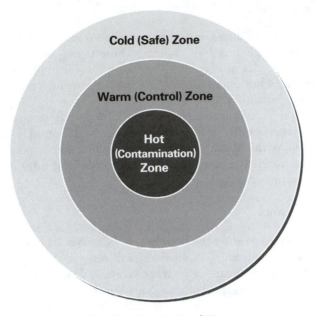

Hot (Contamination) Zone

• Contamination is actually present.
• Personnel must wear appropriate protective gear.
• Number of rescuers limited to those absolutely necessary.
• Bystanders never allowed.

Warm (Control) Zone

• Area surrounding the contamination zone.
• Vital to preventing spread of contamination.
• Personnel must wear appropriate protective gear.
• Life-saving emergency care and decontamination are performed.

Cold (Safe) Zone

• Normal triage, stabilization, and treatment are performed.
• Rescuers must shed contaminated gear before entering the cold zone.

Figure 7-1 Zones of contamination.

The principles of hazmat zone establishment can be applied to all NBC incidents. However, unlike most ordinary hazmat incidents, NBC attacks can frequently be expected to have very large hot zones (many city blocks) and huge warm zones (perhaps the entire city). Rescue workers who ordinarily would not be expected to participate in hazmat operations may find themselves in a potentially contaminated zone owing to the sheer magnitude and incredible potency of an NBC release.

Hazardous Materials Teams

Hazardous materials teams are specialized units that train extensively to safely handle all types of hazardous material, including NBC agents. These teams are equipped with sophisticated barriers and self-contained breathing apparatus capable of protecting workers in the highly contaminated hot zone (Figure 7-2). This equipment is also very effective in chemical or biological situation.

Hazmat teams take an *all hazards* approach when dealing with an unknown hazardous material, such as might be the case early in an NBC incident. This approach assumes the worst and requires the hazmat team to wear maximum protection. It assures safety when the hazardous material is very toxic. If the material later turns out to be a lesser threat, protective measures can be downgraded.

EMS and Medical Personnel

Not all workers will be expected to enter the hot zone. In fact, most EMS providers will not operate in this area at all. Instead, EMS providers will generally work in the warm zone in triage or decontamination teams, or in the cold zone. The level of protection necessary in the warm zone is not as great as that required in the hot zone. Nonetheless,

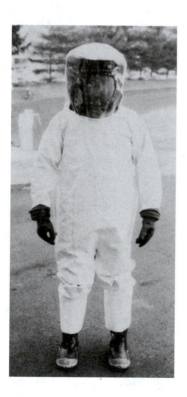

Figure 7-2 Level A suit with self-contained breathing apparatus and fully-encapsulated suit.

specialized and properly fitted equipment is essential for safe operations in this zone. Because all EMS providers may find themselves in a WMD incident, it is important for you to be trained and equipped to protect yourself.

CHEMICAL PROTECTION

Masks

Since the primary routes of entry for most chemical agents are the mouth, nose, lungs, and eyes, a face mask is a critical component of an NBC protection system. The best protection comes from self contained breathing apparatus (SCBA), which is integral in level A and B hazmat protection (Figure 7-3). (The level refers to standard Environmental Protection Agency degrees of protection, with level A being the highest and level D the lowest.) SCBA means the rescuer brings his or her own supply of fresh air. This type of PPE is costly and requires extensive training, so it is usually reserved for use by hazmat technicians in the hot zone. An obvious disadvantage of SCBA is the need to replenish air tanks at frequent intervals.

A lesser but still highly effective degree of protection against NBC agents is the filtering mask. These masks use a combination superactivated charcoal and micropore filtering systems, and are part of level C protection systems (Figure 7-4). Typical masks in common use are listed in Table 7-1. All provide excellent protection against all known chemical and biological agents and airborne fallout when properly donned and worn. Maintaining a good seal is crucial to the effectiveness of the mask. An obvious advantage of the mask is that there is no need to constantly replace the heavy air bottles as in the SCBA systems. A disadvantage of filtering masks is that they will not protect against all hazardous vapors, such as some corrosive substances used in industry, and will not work in oxygen-deficient atmospheres.

Protective Garments

A mask alone is not sufficient protection against some agents, particularly nerve and vesicant agents. Complete protection requires a suitable garment or suit and includes gloves and boots. Two main types are available, the military overgarment and the civilian-style impervious cloth suit. Both provide excellent protection against splashes from all known chemical and biological agents. The military overgarment (Figure 7-5) is a charcoal-imbedded, liquid repellent material. The civilian version is made of waterproof or water repellent cloth such as Dupont Tyvex. The military overgarment has the advantage of being breathable and durable, with a wear time of thirty days in an uncontaminated environment. Vinyl boots and hood and butyl rubber gloves complete the protective ensemble. The Tyvex suit is less expensive, easier to store and widely available in the commercial market. It is much less durable and does not breath, however. Neither type offers positive pressure (Level A) protection, but both provide proven protection

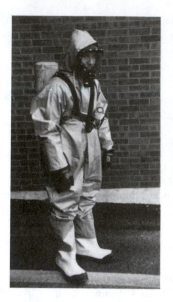
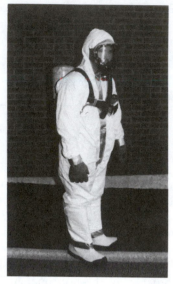
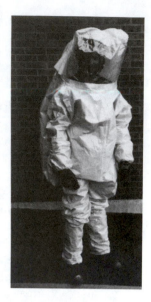

Figure 7-3 Level B suits with self-contained breathing apparatus and chemical-resistant suit.

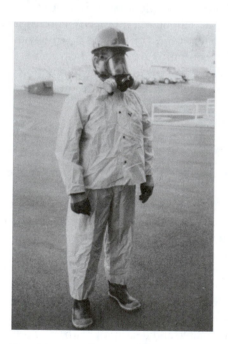
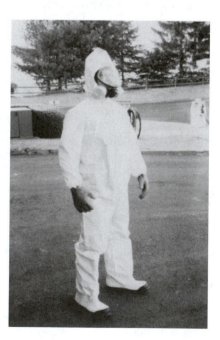

Figure 7-4 Level C suits with respirators and protective garments.

TABLE 7-1

NBC PROTECTION MASKS IN COMMON USE

M17	old-style military mask
M24/25	combat vehicle/aircraft mask
M40/42	newer style field/vehicle mask
Civilian-style	Full-face piece mask
Civilian-style	Half-face price mask

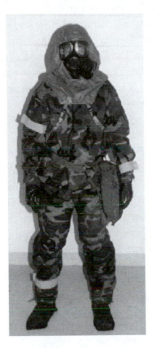

Figure 7-5 Military chemical protective overgarment and M40 mask.

against known chemical and biological threats and alpha radiation. The military over-garment, however, will not protect against many industrial chemicals which the Tyvek suit is resistant to.

Working in Protective Garments

The EMS provider in full NBC protective ensemble will quickly realize the hot, bulky, and cumbersome nature of the gear. Vision and hearing are consequently limited, and manual dexterity is markedly degraded. Heat buildup quickly becomes a problem in all but the coolest conditions. During hot weather, heat exhaustion is a real risk for personnel wearing the ensemble for longer than a few minutes. A rule of thumb is to add 5º-9º C

(10° – 15° F) to the ambient temperature as an estimate of the heat burden when wearing a full suit and mask.

Despite these limitations, it is possible to work and provide adequate medical care when wearing the full protective ensemble. Intubation, starting an intravenous infusion and assessing vital signs are all possible. Certainly, these procedures will take longer than usual to perform. However, careful palpation, auscultation and rechecking of critical findings will improve accuracy and efficiency. Practice drills and simulated patient care are essential training tasks for all EMS providers preparing to treat chemical patients.

Chemical Agent Prophylaxis

Prophylaxis is the use of medications to pretreat individuals not yet exposed but at risk for contact with chemical agents. Pretreatment has the goal of providing some degree of protection against potential chemical threats. The only effective prophylaxis or pretreatment against chemical agents currently available is pyridostigmine. This medication is effective against some types of nerve agents, particularly GD (soman). While pyridostigmine does not offer complete protection against soman, it will improve survival of many exposed individuals. However, it may not be effective against GB (sarin) or VX. Pyridostigmine is not an antidote and should not be administered to patients already exposed to nerve agents, as it can worsen symptoms.

Pyridostigmine is taken every 8 hours whenever the risk of nerve agent exposure is high. The drug causes side effects (mainly vomiting, diarrhea and urinary frequency) in up to 50% of those taking the regimen. However, it is usually well tolerated in healthy adults, and less than 1% will need to discontinue the medication. Thousands of US troops received the regimen during the Gulf War, and pyridostigmine was speculated to be a factor in the mysterious "Gulf War Syndrome." However, strong data supports the safety of the drug. If a serious risk of nerve agent exposure is imminent, the benefits of pyridostigmine pretreatment far outweigh any possible risk.

BIOLOGICAL PROTECTION

Self-protection against biological agents is highly achievable, and all EMS providers should be familiar with these measures. Fortunately, all of the techniques used to protect workers from chemical agents are also very effective for biological agents. The EMS provider need only be familiar with one set of techniques for both biological and chemical agents. The following paragraphs will serve to amplify important points peculiar to biological agent protection.

Protective Mask

Since most biological agents enter the body through the mouth, nose, and lungs, a properly fitted and maintained protective mask is a crucial element in biological self-protection. If a standard NBC mask is not available and the agent is known to be biological, then a medical high-efficiency particulate air (HEPA, OSHA N95) filter will offer limited protection. Many of these masks do not protect the eyes or the rest of the body. To complete the protection, a garment, boots and gloves are also needed.

Protective Garments

Intact skin affords good barrier protection against most biological agents. Nonetheless, a protective garment is essential until safety can be assured. This includes the use of water repellent or waterproof hood, gloves, and boots.

Immunization and Prophylaxis

Perhaps the best protection against biological weapons is prevention. A key tool in preventing any disease is immunization or prophylaxis. Immunization involves taking substances related to the biological agent (but nontoxic and noninfectious) to develop resistance or antibodies. Immunizations are available against many biological agent threats. Prophylaxis is the taking of antibiotics prior to exposure. It can be effective in conjunction with intelligence reports which pinpoint the agent and timing of an attack. Several effective immunizations and prophylaxis strategies are available. The most notable is the anthrax vaccine, which may be up to 95% effective and is relatively free of side effects. Other immunizations and prophylactic antibiotics are administered only when the threat is high. Chapter 5, Care of Biological Agent Illnesses and Table 5-8 list several common preventive strategies against biologic agents.

RADIOLOGICAL PROTECTION

Protection from high intensity radiation (thermal radiation from a nuclear fireball and gamma rays) requires extensive structural shielding and is discussed in Chapter 6, Care of Nuclear Injuries. Protection from the lesser threats of fallout, alpha and gamma radiation is possible using standard protective ensembles as described for chemical agents. No special equipment beyond this NBC ensemble is needed for low-level contamination, but high energy radioactivity will easily penetrate this protection.

Radiologic Prophylaxis

Prophylaxis against one aspect of radioactive contamination, radioactive iodine is possible. A nuclear byproduct, radioactive iodine enters the food chain, and becomes concentrated in the thyroid. Thyroid cell damage caused by this concentration and radioactive decay may lead to an increased incidence of cancer. Administration of nonradioactive iodine to saturate the organ reduces any radiation concentration, and hence reduces the risk of thyroid cancer. Unit (single) dose tablets of sodium iodine are taken orally, once per day. The risk from radioactive iodine lasts for a few weeks, during which time you may be asked to distribute or administer the tablets. Unfortunately, iodide administration does not offer any protection against the many other ill effects of radiation.

Patient Decontamination

Patients exposed to chemical, biologic, or radiologic agents will need to be decontaminated before being allowed to enter the evacuation or transport system. Failure to properly decontaminate the patient may result in dangerous agents being carried into areas where personnel are not be wearing protective ensembles. This places the medical team and others at risk. Furthermore, failing to adequately decontaminate allows greater potential exposure of the patient to hazardous agents. Thorough and rapid decontamination is a critical medical skill for all EMS providers. The principles of NBC decontamination parallel routine hazmat principles practiced by all emergency services and are easily learned.

This section will focus on decontamination provided in the field. Only a general outline will be provided in this section. Readers interested in further details of patient decontamination should consult the references at the end of the chapter. The key considerations in patient decontamination are listed in Table 7-2 and will be briefly outlined.

Wind Direction and Site Selections

Choose a site on relatively high ground that slopes toward and is upwind of the contaminated zone. These measures will reduce the spread of hazardous materials from the contaminated zone (hot or dirty side) to the uncontaminated zone (cold or clean side). If available, establish wastewater collection procedures to reduce environmental contamination.

Security and Control of the Site

Security and control of the site are necessart to keep personnel from inadvertently tracking contamination to the uncontaminated side. Establish a "hot line" boundary between the dirty (contaminated) and clean (decontaminated) sides (Figure 7-6). All personnel on the dirty side must be in full protective ensemble. Personnel on the clean side but close to the hot line should be in protective ensemble as well.

TABLE 7-2

KEY CONSIDERATIONS IN PATIENT DECONTAMINATION

Wind direction and site selection
Security and control of the side
Waste water and contaminated material collection and disposal
Adequate litter patient decontamination
Expeditious ambulatory patient decontamination

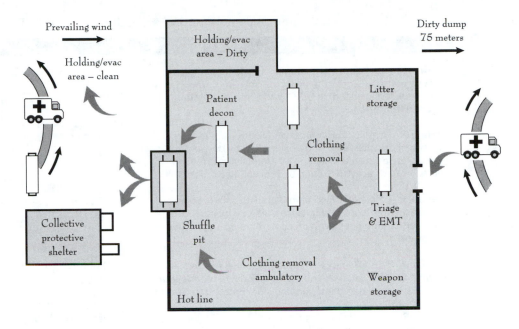

Figure 7-6 Diagram of decontamination station.

TABLE 7-3

OPTIMAL DECONTAMINATION STAGES

1. Physical removal
2. Wet decon (soap and water)
3. Technical decon (decontamination solution)
4. Wet decon (water rinse)

Decontamination Stages

Optimally, NBC decontamination is carried out in four stages (Table 7-3). First is physical removal of the agent, followed by soap and water (dish detergent is adequate), technical decontamination and a final rinse.

Garment Removal

An important first step in patient decontamination is removal of gross contamination, followed by careful removal of all garments (protective and underclothes) except the mask

9-Station Decontamination Procedure

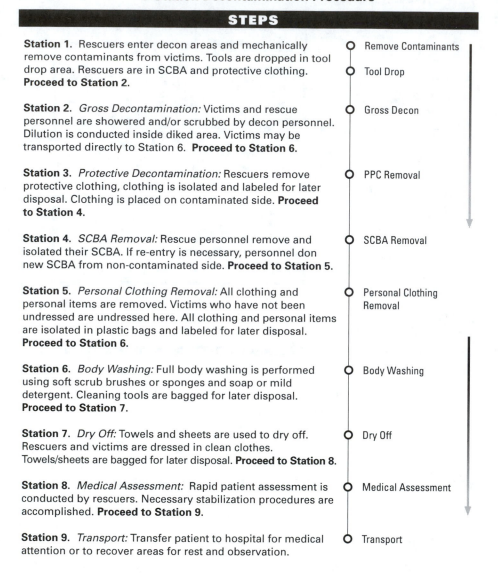

STEPS

Station 1. Rescuers enter decon areas and mechanically remove contaminants from victims. Tools are dropped in tool drop area. Rescuers are in SCBA and protective clothing. **Proceed to Station 2.**

○ Remove Contaminants

○ Tool Drop

Station 2. *Gross Decontamination:* Victims and rescue personnel are showered and/or scrubbed by decon personnel. Dilution is conducted inside diked area. Victims may be transported directly to Station 6. **Proceed to Station 6.**

○ Gross Decon

Station 3. *Protective Decontamination:* Rescuers remove protective clothing, clothing is isolated and labeled for later disposal. Clothing is placed on contaminated side. **Proceed to Station 4.**

○ PPC Removal

Station 4. *SCBA Removal:* Rescue personnel remove and isolated their SCBA. If re-entry is necessary, personnel don new SCBA from non-contaminated side. **Proceed to Station 5.**

○ SCBA Removal

Station 5. *Personal Clothing Removal:* All clothing and personal items are removed. Victims who have not been undressed are undressed here. All clothing and personal items are isolated in plastic bags and labeled for later disposal. **Proceed to Station 6.**

○ Personal Clothing Removal

Station 6. *Body Washing:* Full body washing is performed using soft scrub brushes or sponges and soap or mild detergent. Cleaning tools are bagged for later disposal. **Proceed to Station 7.**

○ Body Washing

Station 7. *Dry Off:* Towels and sheets are used to dry off. Rescuers and victims are dressed in clean clothes. Towels/sheets are bagged for later disposal. **Proceed to Station 8.**

○ Dry Off

Station 8. *Medical Assessment:* Rapid patient assessment is conducted by rescuers. Necessary stabilization procedures are accomplished. **Proceed to Station 9.**

○ Medical Assessment

Station 9. *Transport:* Transfer patient to hospital for medical attention or to recover areas for rest and observation.

○ Transport

Figure 7-7 An example of a field decontamination sequence.

(Figure 7-7). Care must be taken to avoid touching the outer portions of clothing to the patient's skin when removing garments, to avoid contaminating the patient. Appendix B outlines the military approach to garment removal and decontamination of NBC casualties. It provides a useful starting point for designing a local decontamination procedure.

Physical Removal

Liquid and solid agent residue on skin, clothing and equipment is the greatest hazard. Therefore, the primary focus of decontamination is physical removal of the offending agent. Use whatever means are available under the circumstances (Table 7-4). A field-expedient method is to simply use a stick or tree branch to scrape as much of the visible agent off as possible. Copious amounts of water are extremely effective, as would be supplied a low-pressure fire hose or industrial decontamination shower. Smaller amounts of water may be used, but only with great care. There is a risk of a counterproductive effect because it may spread contamination if not completely washed away. This method is less practical if tens of thousands of people require decontamination, owing to the prohibitive volumes of water necessary. If this method is used, care must be taken to control wastewater and avoid further environmental contamination.

Another method of physically removing a chemical agent is to absorb it into a substance such as Fuller earth, a clay-based, highly absorbent quarry product. A generous handful of Fuller earth is rubbed briskly over outer garments or skin. This process is repeated until all surfaces are covered. Careful disposal of the Fuller earth follows. Diatomaceous earth is a similar substance and is an acceptable alternative. Both are widely available from commercial sources and are inexpensive. If possible, use copious amounts of water to thoroughly wash all body surfaces of the patient. A low-pressure fire hose or power cleaner is ideal, as it is able to deliver many gallons of water per minute. When water or other methods of physical removal are not available, the EMS provider must rely on decontamination solutions (discussed later) to neutralize the agent residue.

Radiation Decontamination

Decontaminate casualties once you are remote from the scene and from radioactive fall-out exposure. Bring the contaminated patient to the decontamination site and remove, bag, and set aside the clothing for proper cleaning or disposal. This removes 90 to 95% of external contamination. Then gently wash exposed areas such as the face and hands with soap and water. If water is in short supply, wipe them clean. Irrigate any contaminated wounds or burns with sterile saline or water, if available. Finally, wash and/or clip

---

TABLE 7-4

SOME METHODS OF PHYSICALLY REMOVING CHEMICAL AGENT FROM SKIN AND CLOTHING

METHOD	NOTES
Removal with stick or tree branch	Field expedient method
Copious water irrigation	Large amounts needed
Fuller earth	Absorbs chemical agent
Diatomaceous earth	Substitute for Fuller earth
Borax powder	Dessicates thickened chemical agents and biologicals
Baking soda	Absorbs chemical agent, neutralizes G-series nerve agents

the hair to remove any remaining contamination. Then scan the patient with a Geiger counter. Once decontaminated, the patient presents no further hazard to care personnel.

During the decontamination process, do not vigorously scrub the patient. This may abrade the skin and open a route for infection. Since radiation exposure affects the body's immune system, an injury may become seriously infected or permit infectious agents to invade the body. During the decontamination process, use stretchers that are easily cleaned. Be sure the decontamination process does not move contamination into the patient care area. Contain any waste water and other contaminated material, then dispose of it safely.

Chemical and Biological Decontamination

A highly effective chemical and biological decontamination material is readily available in hypochlorite solution (Table 7-5). It will neutralize virtually all known chemical and biological warfare agents and is thus sometimes termed the "universal decontaminant." Several minutes (up to ten to fifteen minutes) of contact are necessary for the hypochlorite to adequately neutralize chemical agents, however. Do not rinse or remove the hypochlorite solution before this time has elapsed.

Make the hypochlorite solution fresh for each group of patients, as the activity rapidly diminishes over several hours. The 0.5% solution is used on all patient skin surfaces and the protective mask. The 5% solution is used on all garments and equipment (except the mask). Avoid getting either solution in the eyes. Copious normal saline is the decontamination solution of choice for the eyes. Lactated Ringer solution and plain water are acceptable substitutes if saline is unavailable.

If available, copious water (e.g., garden hose) can be used to rinse the patient after using the hypochlorite solutions. Civilian experience has shown that low-pressure power

TABLE 7-5

MAKING DECONTAMINATION SOLUTIONS

5% hypochlorite	Add 8 six-ounce containers of calcium hypochlorite (HTH) to 5 gal water
	or
	Household bleach straight from bottle
0.5% hypochlorite	Add 1 six-ounce container of HTH to 5 gal water
	or
	Add 64 fluid oz (half gal) of bleach to 5 gal water
10% chloramine	Add 3 parts household bleach to 1 part household ammonia Note: fumes are toxic and flammable

cleaners are very effective in decontamination procedures and should be employed when available to supplement the hypochlorite rinses.

If it is known for certain that the agent is a V-series nerve or mustard agent, a chloramine solution may be used to decontaminate equipment (not personnel). Use chloramine solution with care as the fumes are both toxic and flammable.

Litter Patient Decontamination

Once brought to the decontamination station, litter patients should be transferred to a decontaminable litter. The patient is then decontaminated. Care is taken to not break the mask seal during the process.

Ambulatory Patient Decontamination

Patients able to walk are segregated to a separate decontamination line. They, too, are systematically decontaminated, but the sequence is slightly different than for litter patients.

Military Decontamination

The current portable mainstay of military individual decontamination consists of two kits, the M291 and M258. Both kits contain wipes designed to remove chemical agents from the skin and protective equipment and to neutralize these agents. The M258 is the older of the two kits and is being phased out. The active ingredients are caustic and work by alkaline hydrolysis. The M291 is newer, and contains highly adsorbent activated charcoal and resin, which destroys the chemical agents. Both kits are effective for a wide variety of liquid agents and are safe for use on skin or equipment. Care must be taken, however, to avoid contacting the eyes or mouth with decontamination material. EMS providers should consider carrying one of these kits on their person when conducting NBC operations.

DETECTION AND MONITORING

Chemical Detection

Since you cannot feel, see or smell most chemical agents, you will need to rely on specialized equipment to detect, identify and monitor them. A wide variety of detection equipment is potentially available to the hazardous materials team to help in identifying the offending NBC agent. Specialized photo-ionization and spectroscopy devices can pinpoint virtually any known chemical. These devices are very expensive, fragile, and require training to operate and interpret. Only the most advanced hazmat teams have these devices readily available. Instead, most hazmat teams and EMS providers will rely on military equipment to detect suspected chemical agents. Devices such as colorimetric paper and testing kits identify liquid agents (Table 7-6). A handheld device called the Chemical Agent Monitor (CAM) is used by many active, reserve and National Guard

TABLE 7-6

MILITARY CHEMICAL AGENT DETECTION DEVICES

DEVICE	Notes
M8 paper	Detects liquid nerve or vesicant agent • Yellow indicates G series nerve agent • Olive/black indicates V series nerve agent • Red indicates vesicant agent
M9 paper	Similar to M8 paper, but has adhesive backing for application to outer garments and equipment
M256 kit	Colometric kit that can detect both liquid and vapor agents • Tube 1 indicates if vesicant, cyanide or nerve agent is present • Tube 2 indicates if G or V series nerve agent is present • Tube 3 indicates if sulfur mustard is present • Tube 4 indicates if phosgene oxime is present • Tube 5 indicates if hydrogen cyanide or cyanogen is present • Tube 6 indicates low concentration of cyanide
CAM	Chemical Agent Monitor can detect nerve and vesicant agents. • Older models must be manually switched to detect nerve or vesicant agents. • Field CAM (FCAM) switches automatically. • Improved CAM (ICAM) can differentiate between different types of nerve and vesicant agents.

military units and can detect most important chemical agent vapors (Table 7-6). Needless to say, proper training and experience are essential for reliable use of this equipment. All EMS personnel who may treat chemical patients must be familiar with it, but the use and maintenance of these supplies is beyond the scope of this textbook. Interested readers are referred to the military sources listed at the end of this chapter.

Biological Detection

Currently, there is no portable equipment for EMS use that can reliably detect biologic agents in the field. Fixed laboratories such as state health labs and Centers for Disease Control laboratories can play a key role in identifying biological agents in a WMD attack. However, this sophisticated laboratory support takes time and is not immediately available during the initial states of care. In the future, the military may field a number of sophisticated tools to provide rapid detection and identification of biological agents, and EMS providers are encouraged to stay abreast of new developments in this rapidly changing field. In the meantime, the EMS provider will need to rely on knowledge of signs and symptoms of biological agent disease to detect an attack.

Radiological Detection

Since you cannot feel, hear, smell, or see nuclear radiation, you must use a special monitor. This device, called a Geiger counter, measures electrical discharges as ionizing radiation passes through the detection chamber. (The chamber cover blocks all but gamma radiation. Removing it will evaluate the alpha and beta dose). The Geiger counter's electronics then register a radiation exposure level, converted to a dosage per hour rate. This radiologic monitoring will help you define the hazard boundary, determine exposure levels, and suggest special actions such as rescue, evacuation, sheltering, or decontamination as necessary.

Radiation exposure rates vary greatly. The detonation sends several hundreds or thousands of gray (a standardized radiation energy unit) out over the first minute within one to two thousand meters from ground zero. A rapid dose of 300 gray will ultimately result in 50% mortality of those irradiated, and produce the nausea, fatigue, and possible vomiting associated with serious radiation exposure. The radiation released from fallout arrives much more slowly and requires twice the dosage to cause the same damage. Any radiation exposure is cumulative (dosage rate per hour times the hours of exposure).

For most operations, the evacuation threshold occurs whenever the expected cumulative dose will reach 1 rem. Elective lifesaving or rescue actions may expose care providers to as much as 25 rem.

In addition to Geiger counter monitoring, all personnel on the nuclear battlefield or at a detonation or incident should wear personal dosimeters. These "pen-like" devices record the accumulation of radiation and can be read optically. The device provides a measure of the victim's exposure and may suggest when they should be evacuated or moved to shelter. While dosimeters do not record the rate of exposure, their information, especially when combined with that of several casualties, can be very valuable in determining the overall exposure from the incident or detonation. It is important that these devices are read frequently when personnel may be exposed to radiation.

PATIENT CARE IN A CONTAMINATED ENVIRONMENT

Undoubtedly, caring for patients in a contaminated environment will be a challenge. Not only must the EMS provider wear a cumbersome protective ensemble, so too must the patient. This will naturally limit the degree and sophistication of care provided. Nonetheless, lifesaving care can occur in this circumstance. Three special pieces of equipment are available from the military to aid the EMS provider in caring for patients in contaminated environments: 1) the patient protective wrap, 2) the decontaminable litter, and 3) resuscitation device individual chemical (RDIC).

The patient protective wrap is a sleeping bag-like disposable wrap designed to be placed around a patient once he or she is stripped of their overgarments and underclothes. The wrap is permeable to oxygen and carbon dioxide to allow the patient to breath. It is designed to be used on a litter, but can be used as a field-expedient litter by itself if necessary. Patients can spend up to six hours in the wrap.

The decontaminable litter resembles an ordinary military folding litter, but is specially designed to allow thorough patient and litter decontamination. The RDIC is essentially a bag-valve mask filled with a chemical/biologic filter to allow positive pressure ventilation of intubated patients. It is used in the same way as a standard bag-valve mask device.

SUMMARY

Chemical agents pose a serious potential threat to EMS providers. However, with proper training and equipment, it is possible to operate in a chemically-contaminated environment. Familiarization with protective equipment will enable the EMS provider to provide emergency care in contaminated environments with less risk to himself or herself.

FOR FURTHER READING

Medical Management of Chemical Patients, 2d ed. U.S. Army Medical Research Institute of Chemical Defense, Aberdeen Proving Grounds, MD. 1995

Field Manual 3-5 NBC Decontamination. Department of the Army, Washington, DC, 1993

Field Manual 3-4 NBC Protection. Department of the Army, Washington, DC 1992

Field Manual 8-285, Treatment of Chemical Agent Patients and Conventional Military Chemical Patients. Department of the Army, Washington, DC, 1995

Field Manual 8-9, NATO Handbook on Medical Aspects of NBC Defensive Operations. Department of the Army, Washington, DC, 1996

Emergency Response to Terrorism: Basic Concepts Student Manual. US Fire Administration, National Fire Academy. Emmitsburg, MD, 1997

McCaughey BG, et al: Combat casualties in conventional and chemical warfare environment. Military Medicine 1988; 153: 227-229

Danon YL, et al (eds): Chemical Warfare Medicine. Gefen Publishing House, Ltd. Jerusalem, 1994

Spiers EM: Chemical and Biological Weapons. St. Martin's Press. New York, 1984

Zajtchuk R, et al (eds): Medical Aspects of Chemical and Biological Warfare. Department of the Army, Office of the Surgeon General, Washington, DC, 1997

Borak J, et al: Hazardous Materials Exposure. Prentice-Hall, Englewood Cliffs, NJ, 1991

Appendix A

MEDICATIONS

Drugs Listed

1. Albuterol (Ventolin)
2. Amyl Nitrite
3. Atropine
4. Diazepam (Valium)
5. Pralidoxime (2-pam-chloride)
6. Pyridostigmine
7. Sodium Iodine
8. Sodium Nitrite
9. Sodium Thiosulfate

MEDICATION USE

The prescription medications listed in this appendix are for use by properly trained paramedics and other advanced-level providers under the close supervision of a medical director. Specific written protocols are an important aspect of prehospital drug administration and their use is strongly encouraged.

The medications listed were chosen because of their particular significance to the emergency care of weapons of mass destruction incidents. Other important medications are needed to effectively treat many emergencies not peculiar to this setting. Readers are encouraged to review one of the many fine paramedic-level EMT textbooks available for a complete discussion of emergency drugs used in general prehospital practice.

It is the responsibility of all medical providers, including EMS personnel, to use medications in an appropriate and safe manner. While every effort has been made to ensure accuracy of doses and other aspects of pharmacology, this text is in no way intended as a guide for drug administration. All EMS personnel must follow thier local medical protocols when using any medication.

Albuterol (Ventolin, Proventil)

Class: Beta-2 agonist
Description: Sympathomimetic that is selective for Beta-2 adrenergic receptors
Mechanism of action: Stimulates smooth muscle of airway to cause bronchodilation
Indications: Relief of bronchoconstriction caused by pulmonary or riot control chemical agents; also indicated for bronchoconstriction due to asthma, anaphylaxis, chronic lung disease
Contraindications: Known hypersensitivity to albuterol
Precautions: Always monitor the patient's vital signs when administering albuterol. Use with caution in elderly persons or patients with known ischemic heart disease. Auscultate breath sounds before and after treatment.
Side effects: anxiety, nervousness, tachycardia, palpitations, dizziness, headache, dysrhythmias, hypertension, nausea and vomiting
Interactions: Simultaneous use with other sympathomimetics may increase incidence of side effects. Beta-blockers may blunt or completely negate the effects of albuterol.
Dosage: 2.5 mg (0.5 ml of a 0.5% solution) mixed in 5 ml normal saline nebulized A metered dose inhaler (MDI) delivers 90 g of albuterol in each puff. Administer 2 puffs per dose. Dosing can be repeated every 20 min up to 3 doses. For long evacuation, repeat this dosing protocol every 3-4 hours if needed.
Pediatric Dosage: 0.15 mg (0.03 ml)/kg in 2.5-5 ml normal saline nebulized
How Supplied: Solution for nebulization is supplied in single-dose vials containing 2.5 mg (0.5 ml) albuterol. MDIs contain approximately 300 90 g puffs.

Amyl Nitrite

Class: cyanide antidote; nitrite
Description: Reducing agent that converts hemoglobin to methemoglobin Methemoglobin preferentially binds cyanide
Mechanism of Action: Forms methemoglobin in blood by reducing hemoglobin
Indications: Cyanide poisoning with severe symptoms
Contraindications: IV established and able to give sodium nitrite
Precautions: May cause life-threatening methemoglobinemia. A potential drug of abuse, it must be properly secured.
Side Effects: Hypotension, vasodilation, euphoria.
Interactions: May potentiate methemoglobin formation when used with sodium nitrite.
Dosage: 1 ampule crushed and inhaled
Pediatric Dosage: same
How Supplied: A component of the Pasadena Cyanide antidote kit It is not available in all kits supplied to the military.

Atropine

Class: anticholinergic

Description: Parasympatholytic (anticholinergic) that is derived from *Atropa belladonna* plant

Mechanism of Action: A potent anticholinergic that acts by blocking acetylcholine receptors, thus inhibiting parasympathetic stimulation It is an important antidote for nerve agent and organophosphate insecticide poisoning.

Indications: Nerve agent poisoning cardiac arrest, hemodynamically significant bradycardia, and organophosphate poisoning

Contraindications: none for emergencies

Precautions: The traditional maximum dose of 0.4 mg/kg (approximately 3 mg for an adult) may need to be exceeded in nerve agent poisoning. Life-threatening heat stroke may result if given in very hot climates because atropine inhibits sweating.

Side Effects: Blurred vision, dilated pupils, dry mouth, tachycardia, drowsiness and confusion

Interactions: None in the tactical setting

Dosage: For nerve agent poisoning and mild symptoms; 2 mg IV/IM For severe symptoms, 6 mg IV/IM/ET May be repeated in 2 mg increments for a total of 12 mg until secretions are dry. During prolonged evacuation, redose 2 mg every five min up to 20 mg total or until secretions dry

Pediatric Dosage: 0.02 mg/kg (0.1 mg minimum dose)

How supplied: Available in autoinjector form (Mark I) containing atropine 2 mg. Also available in prefilled syringes for IV/IM use containing 1 mg atropine in 10 ml solution

Diazepam (Valium)

Class: Anticonvulsant, sedative

Description: Benzodiazepine which is used as an anticonvulsant and sedative

Mechanism of Action: Suppresses the spread of seizure activity across the brain Does not appear to suppress the seizure focus Induces sedation and muscle relaxation by directly stimulating specific brain receptors

Indications: Convulsions associated with nerve agents Also used to stop other seizures, and as a sedating and anti-anxiety agent for cardioversion and other painful or uncomfortable procedures

Contraindications: Known hypersensitivity to diazepam

Precautions: Diazepam is a relatively short-acting drug. During prolonged evacuation, seizures may recur. Injectable diazepam is irritating to veins, so use the largest IV catheter possible when administering by IV. A controlled substance, it must be properly secured Diazepam can be reversed with flumazenil (Romazicon).

Side Effects: Hypotension, drowsiness, headache, amnesia, respiratory depression, blurred vision, nausea and vomiting

Interactions: Diazepam is incompatible with many medications. Any time diazepam is given intravenously, be sure to flush the line before and after administration. The effect of diazepam can be additive with other CNS depressants and alcohol.

Dosage: For convulsions associated with nerve agent poisoning 10 mg IV/IM/ET. May be repeated in 5 mg increments every 5 minute up to 20 mg or until convulsions stop.

For prolonged evacuation, dose 10 mg every 2-3 hours as needed to control seizures.

Pediatric Dosage: 0.2 mg/kg IV/IM/ET up to 10 mg.

How Supplied: Available as autoinjector containing diazepam 10 mg. Also available in ampules and prefilled syringes containing 10 mg in 2 ml solvent

Note: Other benzodiazepines such as lorazepam (Ativan) are equally effective in controlling seizures. Substitution (at the appropriate dose) is permissible if authorized by a physician.

Pralidoxime (Protopam, 2-Pam-Chloride)

Class: Oxime

Description: Regenerator of acetylcholinesterase (AChE) that has been inactivated by a nerve agent or organophosphate insecticide

Mechanism of Action: Breaks the bond between the nerve agent and AChE, thus restoring its function

Indications: Nerve agent poisoning

Contraindications: None in emergencies

Precautions: Will variably regenerate AChE depending on the type of nerve agent and the time elapsed since exposure. Some nerve agents age with time (minutes to hours) and become resistant to pralidoxime effects.

Side Effects: Inconsequential in the setting of nerve agent poisoning

Interactions: Works synergistically with atropine and the two should always be used together.

Dosage: For mild symptoms, 600 mg IV/IM. For severe symptoms 1800 mg IV/IM For prolonged evacuation, redosing may be required at 1000 mg IV/IM every 60 min over 20 minutes or until spontaneous respirations return.

Pediatric Dosage: For mild symptoms, 25 mg/kg up to 600 mg. IV/IM For severe symptoms 50 mg/kg up to 1 gm IV/IM. For prolonged transport, redosing may be required at 15 mg/kg IV/IM every 60 min over 20 minutes or until spontaneous respirations return.

How Supplied: Available in autoinjector (Mark I) containing pralidoxime 600 mg. Also available in vials containing 1 gm of powder for reconstitution with 20 ml sterile water

Pyridostigmine

Class: Cholinergic-stimulating agent

Description: Carbamate acetylcholinesterase (AChE) inhibitor

Mechanism of Action: Temporarily blocks the enzyme AChE When taken as a pretreatment, pyridostigmine blocks some of the AChE receptors. These blocked receptors are then unavailable for binding with nerve agents. After a few hours, the pyridostigmine releases the AChE, restoring normal function.

Indications: Pretreatment when the risk of nerve agent exposure, particularly soman (GD) is high. May not be effective for sarin (GB) or VX nerve agents

Contraindications: Known hypersensitivity to pyridostigmine. Not an antidote and may worsen nerve agent toxicity and so is contraindicated if exposure has already occurred. Also contraindicated in urinary and gastric obstruction

Precautions: May precipitate severe respiratory distress in asthmatics

Side Effects: Nausea, vomiting, abdominal cramps, salivation, increased bronchial secretions, constricted (pinpoint) pupils, sweating, and skin rash. Can also cause weakness and fasciculations (localized muscle twitching)

Interactions: Effects can be additive if taken with similar medications such as neostigmine or physostigmine. Over time, tablets of pyridostigmine can become mottled from exposure to moisture. This does not affect the medication.

Dosage: 30 mg po every 8 hours

Pediatric Dosage: Not established for pretreatment. However, based on information on the use of pyridostigmine in children for other reasons, a dose of 0.5 mg/kg up to 30 mg po every 8 hours may be effective.

How Supplied: 30 mg tablets in a seven-day (21 tablets) blister-pack Also available as 60 mg scored tablets (half tablet is 30 mg) and in syrup form, 60 mg per 5 ml.

Sodium Iodine

Class: Essential trace element

Description: Trace mineral required by the thyroid gland to produce thyroid hormone

Mechanism of Action: Blocks the uptake of radioactive iodine by the thyroid gland

Indications: When radioactive iodine has been (or there is an imminent threat) released into the air or contaminates the food supply

Contraindications: Known hypersensitivity to sodium iodide

Precautions: none

Side Effects: Possible skin rashes, swelling of the salivary glands, a metallic taste in the mouth, and sore teeth, throat and gums. More severe but very rare effects include fever, joint pain, facial or body swelling, and shortness of breath.

Interactions: None

Dosage: One tablet (130 mg) per day Preferably, start the medication several days before or soon after exposure to radioactive iodine. However, the medication may be given at any time after exposure.

Pediatric Dosage: One table (130 mg) per day for children 1 year and older. Half tablet (65 mg) per day for children under 1-year old Crush tablet and mix with food or drink as needed.

How Supplied: Multi-tablet vial of 130 mg tablets.

Sodium Nitrite

Class: Cyanide antidote; nitrite

Description: Reducing agent that converts hemoglobin to methemoglobin

Mechanism of Action: Forms methemoglobin in blood by reducing hemoglobin. Methemoglobin preferentially binds cyanide.

Indications: Cyanide poisoning with severe symptoms

Contraindications: None in emergencies

Precautions: May cause life-threatening methemoglobinemia

Side Effects: Hypotension, vasodilation, euphoria

Interactions: May potentiate methemoglobin formation when used with amyl nitrite

Dosage: 300 mg IV over 2-4 minutes

Pediatric Dosage: 6-10 mg/kg up to 300 mg IV over 2-4 minutes

How Supplied: Available in Pasadena Cyanide antidote kit as a 10 ml ampule containing 3% sodium nitrite

Sodium Thiosulfate

Class: sulfate-forming compound

Description: A sulfate-forming compound that reacts with cyanide-methemoglobin

Mechanism of Action: Reacts with cyanide-methemoglobin complex in blood to detoxify the cyanide and allow excretion by the kidneys.

Indications: Suspected cyanide poisoning with severe symptoms

Contraindications: Do not administer until after sodium nitrite is administered.

Precautions: Does not detoxify cyanide unless a nitrite (amyl or sodium nitrite) is administered first.

Side Effects: Hypotension is the chief side effect.

Interactions: Works together with nitrites to detoxify cyanide.

Dosage: 12.5 gm IV

Pediatric Dosage: 250-400 mg/kg up to 12.5 gm IV. Use 5 ml of sodium thiosulfate of each ml of sodium nitrite administered.

How Supplied: Available in Pasadena cyanide antidote kit as a 50 ml ampule of 25% sodium thiosulfate

Appendix B

NBC PROTECTION PROCEDURES

Procedures Listed

1. Donning M40 series mask and hood
2. Donning M17 series mask and hood
3. Decontamination using the M258 kit
4. Decontamination using the M291 kit
5. Donning the military chemical protective overgarment
6. Decontamination procedure for litter patient
7. Decontamination procedure for ambulatory patient
8. Administering the Mark I autoinjector

The military has long been recognized as expert in dealing with weapons of mass destruction threats and, in particular, NBC agents. This material is presented to provide the civilian EMS provider with some insight into military procedures for donning personal protective equipment and decontaminating patients. This material is presented for informational purposes only. Civilian EMS providers may have contact with and be working side-by-side with military personnel in a WMD incident. This section will familiarize civilian personnel with various aspects of military NBC procedures.

This information is not intended to be adopted directly by civilian medical providers in a civilian setting. Instead, civilians should look to the agency director, department chief, medical director, hazmat specialist, and to other key personnel for advice and guidance on PPE procedures and patient decontamination procedures. Military equipment has not been recognized and approved by civilian regulatory agencies including the Occupational Safety and Health Administration (OSHA) and the Environmental Protection Agency (EPA). The Mark I autoinjector has similarly not been approved by the Food and Drug Administration for use outside the military setting.

This appendix is adapted from Soldier training Publication STP-21-1-SMCT Soldier's manual of Common Tasks, Department of the Army, Washington, DC, 1994, Medical Management of Chemical Casualties, Medical Research Institute of Chemical Defense, Aberdeen Proving grounds, MD, 1995, Field Manual 8-230, Medical Specialist, Department of the Army, Washington, DC, 1984.

1. Donning M40 Mask and Hood (Figure B-1)

1. Don your mask within 9 seconds.
   a. Stop breathing.
   b. Close your eyes.
   c. Remove your headgear and place your headgear in a convenient location, avoiding contaminated surfaces, if possible.

WARNING

DO NOT WEAR CONTACT LENSES WITH PROTECTIVE MASK. REMOVE CONTACT LENSES WHEN THE USE OF CHEMICAL AGENTS IS IMMINENT.

   d. Take off your glasses, placing them in a safe place.
   e. Open the carrier with your left hand holding the carrier open.
   f. Remove the mask from the carrier by grasping the mask with your right hand.

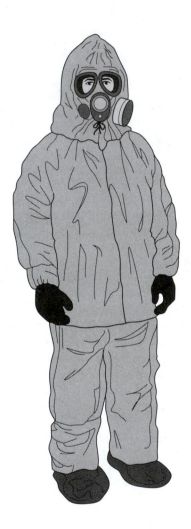

Figure B-1   M40 Mask and hood.

g. Put your chin in the chin pocket.

h. Seal the mask.

(1) Cover the openings at the bottom of the outlet valve with the palm of your hand.

(2) Blow out hard so that air escapes around the edges of the mask.

(3) Cover the inlet port of the canister with the palm of your hand.

(4) Breath in.

Note: The facepiece should collapse against your face and remain so while you hold your breath. If it does, the facepiece is airtight. If the facepiece does not collapse, check for hair, clothing, or other matter between the facepiece and your face.

(5) Remove anything preventing a seal from forming between your face and the mask.

I. Don the head harness.

(1) Pull the head harness over your head after grasping the tab.

(2) Position the harness so that your ears are between the temple straps and the cheek straps.

j. tighten the face straps one at a time with one hand while holding the facepiece to your face with the other hand to maintain the seal.

k. Center the headpad at the high point on the back of your head.

Note: The straps should lie flat against your head.

l. Clear your mask again.

m. Recheck your facepiece for leaks.

n. Resume breathing.

2. Don the hood so that it lies smoothly on your head.

CAUTION

BE VERY CAREFUL WHEN PULLING ON THE HOOD. THE HOOD COULD SNAG ON THE BUCKLES OF THE HEAD HARNESS AND TEAR.

a. Grasp the back edge of the hood skirt.

b. Pull the hood carefully over your head so that it covers the back of your neck, head, and shoulders.

c. Zip the front of the hood closed by pulling the zipper slider downward.

d. Tighten the draw cord.

e. Secure the underarm straps by fastening and adjusting them.

f. Put on your helmet.

g. Close your mask carrier.

h. Continue the mission.

3. Remove your protective mask with hood after the "all clear" order is given.

a. Remove your helmet.

b. Unfasten the underarm straps.

c. Loosen the draw cord.

d. Unzip the zipper on the hood.

4. Continue your mission.

2. Donning M17 Mask and Hood (Figure B-2)

1. Don your mask within 9 seconds.
   a. Stop breathing, holding your breath until the mask is sealed and cleared.
   b. Remove your headgear.
   c. Place your headgear in a convenient location, avoiding contaminated surfaces, if possible.
   d. Remove your glasses, placing them in a safe place (for example, the overgarment pocket), if appropriate.
   e. Open your mask carrier with your left hand holding the carrier open.
   f. Grasp your mask just below the eyepiece with your right hand.
   g. Pull the mask out of the carrier so that the hood hangs inside out in front of the facepiece.
   h. Grasp the facepiece with both hands. (Figure B-3)
   I. Slide your thumbs up and inside the mask, opening the head harness and facepiece as wide as you can.
   j. Put your chin in the chin pocket.
   k. Pull the head harness up over your head, making sure the head pad is centered at the top back of your head and the mask is smooth against your face and forehead.

Note: Never put the head harness over your head first and then pull the mask down over your face.

   l. Adjust the mask by grasping the cheek straps with both hands and pulling them with moderate jerks.
   m. Clear the mask by the following steps:

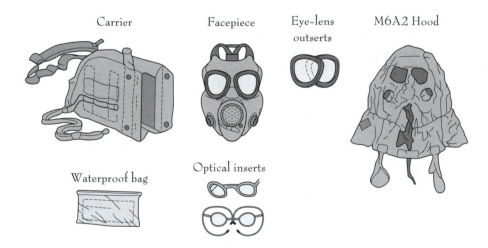

Carrier   Facepiece   Eye-lens outserts   M6A2 Hood

Waterproof bag   Optical inserts

Figure B-2 M17 mask and hood.

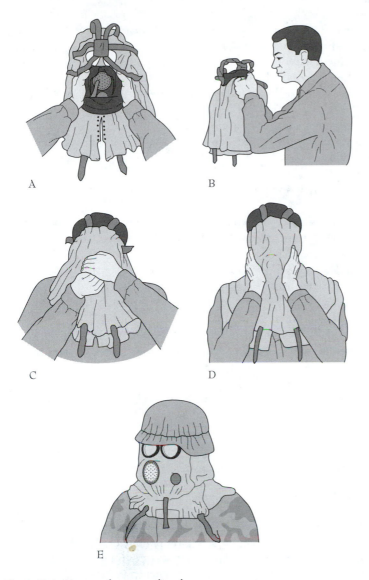

A B C D

E

Figure B-3 Grasping facepiece of mask.

(1) Seal the outlet valve and voicemitter by cupping the heel of one hand over the outlet valve and placing the other hand over the voicemitter and applying pressure.

Note: You can either put your hands over or under the hood to do this.

(2) Blow hard to force air out around the edges of the mask.

n. Check the mask.
   (1) Place the palms of your hands over both inlet valve caps.
   (2) Seal the valves by applying pressure.
Note: you can either put your hands over or under the hood to do this.
   (3) Suck in and hold your breath.
Note: If there are no leaks, your mask will collapse against your face and stay that way until you breath out.
   (a) Go to step 1p, if you find your mask has no leaks.
   (b) Go to step 1o, if your mask does not collapse.
o. Reseat a mask that leaks.
   (1) Stop breathing.
   (2) Check to see if there is anything, such as hair or clothing, between your face and the mask.
   (3) Remove anything that would keep the mask from sealing against your face.
   (4) Make sure the head straps and the head pad are not twisted.
   (5) Tighten the head straps, if necessary.
   (6) Clear your mask by repeating step 1m.
   (7) Recheck your mask for leaks using step 1n.
p. Start breathing normally.
2. Don the hood within an additional 6 seconds.
   a. Pull the hood up and over your head and down onto your shoulders.
   b. Zip the front closed all the way, making sure the edge of the hood does not get caught in the collar of the overgarment.
3. Pull the draw cord slider snug, as the mission allows.
4. Fasten the underarm straps, adjusting them with buddy aid, if available as the mission allows.
5. Replace your headgear.
6. Close your mask carrier.
7. Continue your mission.

3. Decontaminate your skin and personal equipment using an M258A1 decontamination kit

WARNING

THE M258A1 DECONTAMINATION KIT (OLIVE DRAB CASE AND WIPE PACKETS) WILL ONLY BE USED FOR ACTUAL CHEMICAL DECONTAMINATION. DO NOT USE WIPES ON YOUR EYES, MOUTH, OR OPEN WOUNDS. THESE AREAS SHOULD BE FLUSHED WITH WATER. FOR DECONTAMINATION OF BLISTERS GIVE FIRST AID FOR BURNS.

1. Don your mask and hood without-
   a. Zipping the hood.
   b. Pulling the draw strings.
   c. Fastening the shoulder straps.
2. Seek overhead cover or use your poncho for protection against further contamination.
3. Decontaminate your hands with decontaminating wipe.
   a. Open the decontamination kit.

b. Remove one decontaminating 1 packet.

c. Fold the packet on the solid line marked BEND.

d. Unfold the packet.

e. Tear open the packet at the notch.

f. Remove the wipe, fully unfolding it.

g. Wipe your skin, starting with your hands.

4. Decontaminate your eyes, if necessary.

    a. Check your canteen for contamination.

        (1) Remove your canteen.

        (2) Unscrew the cap, avoiding possible contamination of the canteen cap by pushing up on the bottom of the canteen cover until you an grasp the canteen by its body.

        (3) Check the canteen mouth for contamination.

            (a) Obtain an uncontaminated canteen.

            (b) Decontaminate the canteen mouth with M258A1 decontamination kit.

    b. Unseal your mask as follows:

        (1) Hold your breath.

        (2) Close your eyes.

        (3) Lift the hood and mask from your chin.

    c. Flush your eyes with water from the canteen.

        (1) Look up, tilting your head to the side to be decontaminated.

        (2) Keep your eyes open.

        (3) Pour water slowly into your eye without letting the water run onto your clothing.

        (4) Flush the other eye, if necessary, using the same steps.

    d. Secure your mask by—

        (1) Resealing it.

        (2) Clearing it.

        (3) Checking it.

    e. Breathe.

5. Decontaminate your face, if necessary, with a decontaminating wipe 1.

    a. Unseal your mask as follows:

        (1) Hold your breath.

        (2) Close your eyes.

        (3) Lift the hood and mask from your chin.

    b. Wipe up and down from ear to ear.

        (1) Start at your ear.

        (2) Wipe across your face to the corner of your nose.

        (3) wipe across your face to the other ear.

    c. Wipe up and down from your ear to the end of your jawbone.

        (1) Begin where step b ended.

        (2) Wipe across your cheek to the corner of your mouth.

        (3) Wipe across your closed mouth to the center of your upper lip.

        (4) Wipe across your closed mouth to the corner of your mouth.

        (5) Wipe across your cheek to the end of your jawbone.

    d. Wipe up and down from one end of your jawbone to the other end of your jaw-bone.

      (1) Begin where you ended in step c.

      (2) Wipe across and under your jaw to your chin, cupping your chin.

      (3) Wipe across and under your jaw to the end of your jawbone.

    e. Turn your hand out and quickly wipe the inside of the mask that touches your face.

Note: Do not wipe the mask lens. The decontaminating solution may leave a film on the lens.

    f. Secure your mask by-

      (1) Resealing it.

      (2) Clearing it.

      (3) checking it.

    g. Breathe.

6. Decontaminate your neck and ears, if necessary, using the same decontamination 1 wipe.

7. Decontaminate your hands again with the same decontaminating 1 wipe.

8. Properly dispose of the contaminated wipe.

9. Prepare the decontaminating 2 wipe.

    a. Pull out one decontaminating 2 wipe packet.

    b. Crush the enclosed glass ampule between your thumb and fingers without kneading.

    c. Fold the packet on the solid line marked CRUSH AND BEND.

    d. Unfold it.

    e. Tear the packet open quickly at the notch.

    f. Remove the wipe.

    g. Open the wipe fully.

    h. Dispose of the crushed glass ampule by burying it.

10. Repeat steps 5 through 8 using the decontaminating 2 wipe.

11. Put on your protective gloves.

12. Fasten your hood.

13. Make sure all skin areas that you have decontaminated are covered.

14. Decontaminate your personal equipment.

Note: Do not use the decontaminating kit on protective overgarments.

    a. Decontaminate weapons, gloves, helmet, and hand tools using decontaminating 1 wipe first, then decontaminating 2 wipe.

    b. Decontaminate the exterior of the hood and mask.

      (1) Wipe eye lens outserts using a decontaminating 2 wipe.

      (2) Begin wiping the hood at the top working your way downward.

      (3) Repeat (1) and (2) above using decontaminating 1 wipe.

Note: Using the wipes in this order will prevent a residue from forming on the eyelens outserts.

15. Remove radiological contamination from your clothing, equipment, and exposed skin if necessary.

    a. Shake or brush contaminated dust from your clothing, equipment, or exposed skin with a brush, broom, or your hands (if a brush or broom is not available).

b. Wash your body as soon as possible, giving special attention to the hairy areas and underneath your fingernails.

4. Decontaminate your skin using the M291 skin decontaminating kit (SDK)

1. Inspect the M291 SDK for loose black powder.
    a. If no powder is detected, the kit is mission ready.
    b. If powder is detected, inspect each packet for leaks.
    c. Discard all leaking packets.
    d. Reinsert good packets into the carrying pouch.
2. Verify that there are at least four skin decontaminating packets in the kit.
Note: If there are less than four packets, request an additional kit, continuing to use your kit until all packets are gone.
CAUTION
FOR EXTERNAL USE ONLY. MAY BE SLIGHTLY IRRITATING TO THE SKIN OR EYES. KEEP DECONTAMINATING POWDER OUT OF YOUR EYES, CUTS, AND WOUNDS. USE WATER TO WASH TOXIC AGENT OUT OF YOUR EYES, CUTS, OR WOUNDS.
   3. Decontaminate your skin with the M291 SDK within one minute of the suspected exposure.
       a. Put on your mask and hood without -
           (1) Zipping the hood.
           (2) Pulling the draw strings.
           (3) Fastening the shoulder straps.
       b. Seek overhead cover for protection against further contamination.
       c. Remove one skin decontaminating packet from the carrying pouch.
       d. Tear the packet open quickly at the notch.
       e. Remove the applicator pad from the packet.
       f. Properly dispose of the empty packet.
       g. Open the applicator pad.
           (1) Unfold the applicator pad.
           (2) Slip your finger(s) into the handle.
       h. Throughly scrub exposed skin on the back of your hand, palm, and fingers until completely covered with black powder from the applicator pad.
       I. Switch the applicator pad to the other hand, repeating the previous step on the other hand.
WARNING
DEATH OR INJURY MAY RESULT IF YOU BREATHE TOXIC AGENTS WHILE DECONTAMINATING THE FACE. IF YOU NEED TO BREATHE BEFORE YOU FINISH, RESEAL YOUR MASK, CLEAR IT, AND CHECK IT. GET YOUR BREATH, THEN RESUME THE DECONTAMINATING PROCEDURE.
       j. Decontaminate your face and the inside of your mask.
           (1) Hold your breath.
           (2) Close your eyes.
           (3) Grasp the mask beneath your chin.
           (4) Pull the hood and mask away from your chin enough to allow one hand between the mask and your face.

(5) Wipe up and down across your face, beginning at the front of one ear to your nose to other ear.

(6) Wipe across your face to the corner of your nose.

(7) Wipe extra strokes at the corner of your nose.

(8) Wipe across your nose and the tip of your nose to the other corner of your nose.

(9) Wipe extra strokes at the corner of your nose.

(10) Wipe across your face to the other ear.

(11) Wipe up and down across your face, beginning from the ear to your mouth to other end of the jawbone.

(12) Wipe across your cheek to the corner of your mouth.

(13) Wipe extra strokes at the corner of your mouth.

(14) Wipe across your closed mouth to the center of your upper lip.

(15) Wipe extra strokes above your upper lip.

(16) Wipe across your closed mouth to the other corner of your mouth.

(17) Wipe extra strokes at the corner of your mouth.

(18) Wipe across your cheek to the end of your jawbone.

(19) Wipe up and down across your face, beginning from your jawbone, to your chin and to the other end of your jawbone.

(20) Wipe across and under your jaw to your chin, cupping your chin.

(21) Wipe extra strokes at the center of your chin.

(22) Wipe across and under your jaw to end of your jawbone.

(23) Decontaminate the inside of your mask by turning your hand out and quickly wiping the inside of the mask that touches your face.

(24) Properly dispose of the applicator pad.

(25) Seal your mask.

(26) Clear your mask.

(27) Check your mask.

(28) Breathe.

k. Remove the second packet from the carrying pouch.

l. Tear open the packet quickly at the notch.

m. Remove the applicator pad from the packet.

n. Discard the empty packet, employing litter discipline.

o. Open the applicator pad.

    (1) Unfold the applicator pad.

    (2) Slip your finger(s) into the handle.

p. scrub throughly the skin of your neck and ears without breaking the seal between your face and the mask until they are completely covered with black powder.

q. Redo your hands until they are completely covered with black powder.

r. Properly dispose of the applicator pad.

s. Put on your protective gloves.

t. Fasten the hood.

u. Remove the powder with soap and water when operational conditions permit.

Note: It does not matter how long the powder stays on your skin.

5. Donning military chemical protective overgarment

1. Put on an uncontaminated overgarment.
   a. Have your buddy open a package containing a new overgarment without touching the garment itself. (Figure B-4)
   b. Pull out the overgarment one piece at a time without touching the outside of the package.
      (1) Put on the new trousers, leaving the cuffs open.
      (2) Put on the jacket.
2. Put on the overboots. (Figure B-5)
   a. Have your buddy pick up a new package of overboots.
   b. Have your buddy open it without touching the overboots inside.
   c. Reach into the package.
   d. Remove the overboots.
   e. Put the overboots on.
3. Put on the green vinyl overboots (GVOs). (Figure B-5)
   a. have your buddy pick up a new package of GVOs, opening it without touching the GVOs inside.
   b. Reach into the package, removing the GVOs.
   c. Put on the GVOs.

Note: GVO donning procedures are very basic; donning is done just like a regular wet weather boot.

4. Put on the gloves. (Figure B-6)

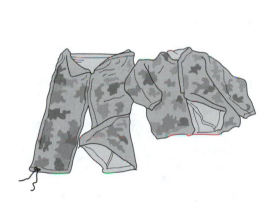

Figure B-4 Uncontaminated overgarment.

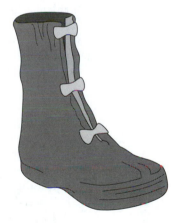

Figure B-5 Overboots.

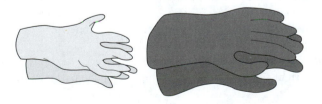

Figure B-6 Gloves.

a. Have your buddy pick up a package of new chemical protective gloves, opening it without touching the gloves inside.

b. Remove the gloves from the package.

c. Put the gloves on.

5. Secure the hood.

a. Have your buddy decontaminate his or her chemical protective gloves with the personal decontamination kit.

b. Have your buddy reposition the hood as follows:

Note: The buddy's gloves must be decontaminated before proceeding with this step.

(1) Unroll your hood.

(2) Reattach the straps.

c. Check all the zippers and ties on your hood and overgarment to ensure they are closed.

6. Repeat steps 3 through 15, taking the role of the buddy.

7. Secure your gear.

a. Place the new chemical protective cover on your helmet.

b. Put your individual gear back on.

c. Check the fit of the secured gear of your buddy.

d. Have him or her check your gear.

6. Decontamination procedure for litter patient

1. Decontaminate the mask and hood: Sponge down front, sides, and top of hood with 5.0% calcium hypochlorite solution, or wipe off with the M258A1 or the M291 Decon Kit.

2. Remove hood

a. Dip scissors in 5% hypochlorite (HTH) solution.

b. Cut off hood. (Figure B-7)

(1) Release or cut hood shoulder straps.

(2) Cut/untie neck cord.

(3) Cut/remove zipper cord.

(4) Cut/remove drawstring under the voicemitter.

(5) Unzip the hood zipper.

(6) Cut the cord away from the mask.

(7) Cut the zipper below voicemitter.

(8) Proceed cutting upward, close to the inlet valve covers and eye lens out-serts.

(9) Cut upward to top of eye lens outsert.

(10) Cut across forehead to the outer edge of the next eye lens outsert.

(11) Cut downward toward patient's shoulder staying close to the eye lens out-sert inlet valve cover.

(12) Cut across the lower part of the voicemitter to the zipper.

(13) Dip scissors in hypochlorite solution.

(14) Cut from center of forehead over the top of the head.

(15) Fold left and right sides of the hood to the side of the patient's head, laying sides on the litter.

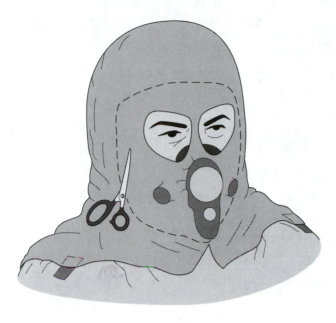

Figure B-7 Cutting off hood.

   c. the Quick Doff Hood is loosened and removed.

3. Decontaminate protective mask/face
   a. Use M258A1, M291, or 0.5% hypochlorite solution.
   b. Cover both inlet valve covers with gauze or hands.
   c. Wipe external parts of mask.
   d. Uncover inlet valve covers.
   e. Wipe exposed areas of patient's face.
     (1) Chin
     (2) Neck
     (3) Back of ears

4. Remove Field Medical Care (FMC) or triage tag
   a. Cut FMC tie wire.
   b. Allow FMC to fall into a plastic bag.
   c. Seal plastic bag and wash with 0.5% hypochlorite.
   d. Place plastic bag under back of mask head straps. (Figure B-8)

5. Remove all gross contamination from patient's overgarment.
   a. Wipe all evident contamination spots with M258A1 Decon Kit, M291, or 5% hypochlorite.
   b. Wipe external parts of mask with M258A1 Decon Kit, or M291.
   c. Use wipe 1 then wipe 2, to clean exterior of mask; use wipe 2 then site 1 to clean interior.

6. Cut and remove overgarments. Cut clothing around tourniquets, bandages, and splints. Two persons will be cutting clothing at the same time. Dip scissors in 5% hypochlorite solution before doing each complete cut to avoid contaminating inner clothing.

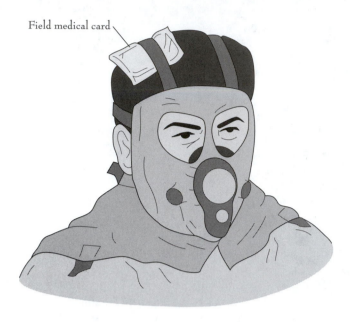

Field medical card

Figure B-8 Place field medical card (in plastic bag) in mask head straps.

    a. Cut overgarment jacket. (Figure B-9)
       (1) Unzip protective overgarment.
       (2) Cut from wrist area of sleeves, up to armpits, and then to neck area.
       (3) Roll chest sections to respective sides with inner surface outward.
       (4) Tuck clothing between arm and chest.
       (5) Repeat procedure for other side of jacket.
    b. Cut overgarment trousers. (Figure B-10)
       (1) Cut from cuff along inseam to waist on left leg.
       (2) On right overgarment leg, cut from cuff to just below zipper and then go sideways into the first cut.
       (3) Allow trouser halves to drop to litter with contamination away from patient.
       (4) Tuck trouser halves to sides of body and roll the camouflage sides under between the legs.
  7. Remove outer gloves. This procedure can be done with one medic on each side of the patient working simultaneously. Do not remove inner gloves. (Figure B-11)
    a. Lift the patient's arms by grasping his gloves.
    b. Fold the glove away from the patient over the sides of the litter.
    c. Grasp the fingers of the glove.
    d. Roll the cuff over the finger, turning the glove inside out.
    e. Carefully lower the arm(s) across the chest when the glove(s) is removed. (Do not allow the arms to contact the exterior (camouflage side) of the overgarment.)
    f. Dispose of contaminated gloves.
       (1) Place in plastic bag.
       (2) Deposit in contaminated dump.
    g. Dip your own gloves in hypochlorite solution.

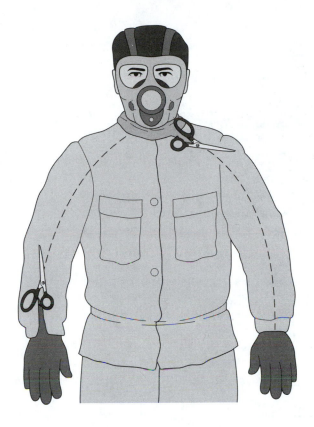

Figure B-9 Cut overgarment jacket.

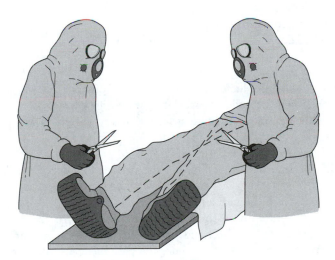

Figure B-10 Cut overgarment trousers.

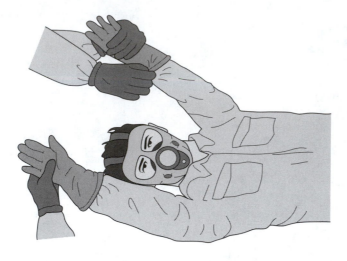

8. Remove overboots.
    a. Hold heels with one hand.
    b. Pull overboots downwards over the heels with other hand.
    c. Pull towards you until removed.
    d. Place overboots in contaminated disposal bag.
9. Remove personal articles from pockets.
    a. Place in plastic bags.
    b. Seal bags.
    c. Place in contaminated holding area.
10. Remove combat boots without touching body surfaces.
    a. Cut boot laces along the tongue.
    b. Pull boots downward and toward you until removed.
    c. Place boots in contaminated dump.
11. Remove inner clothing.
    a. Unbuckle belt.
    b. Cut BDU pants following same procedures as for overgarment trousers.
    c. Cut fatigue jacket following same procedures as for overgarment jacket.
12. Remove undergarments following same procedure as for fatigues. If patient is wearing a brassiere, it is cut between cups. Both shoulder straps are cut where they attach to cups and laid back off shoulders.
13. Clothing removal and skin decontamination: Transfer the patient to a decontamination litter. After the patient's clothing has been cut away, he is transferred to a decontamination litter or a canvas litter with a plastic sheeting cover. Three decontamination team members decontaminate their gloves and apron with the 5% hypochlorite solution. One member places his hands under the small of the patient's legs and thigh; a second member places his arms under the patient's back and buttocks; and the third member places his arms under the patient's shoulders and supports the head and neck. They carefully lift the patient using their knees, not their backs to minimize back strain. While the patient is elevated, another decon team

member removes the litter from the litter stands and another member replaces it with a decontamination (clean) litter. The patient is carefully lowered onto the clean litter. Two decon members carry the litter to the skin decontamination station. The contaminated clothing and overgarments are placed in bags and moved to the decontaminated waste dump. The dirty litter is rinsed with the 5% decontamination solution and placed in a litter storage area. Decontaminated litters are returned to the ambulances.

14. Skin decontamination: The areas of potential contamination should be spot decontaminated using the M258A1 kit, the M291 kit, or 0.5% hypochlorite. These areas include the neck, wrists, lower face, and skin under tears or holes in the protective ensemble. After the patient is deconned his dressings and tourniquet are changed. Superficial (not body cavities, eyes or nervous tissue) wounds are flushed with the 0.5% hypochlorite solution and new dressings applied as needed. Cover massive wounds with plastic or plastic bags. New tourniquets are placed 0.5 to 1 inch proximal to the original tourniquet, then the old tourniquets are removed. Splints are not removed but saturated to the skin with 0.5% hypochlorite solution. If the splint cannot be saturated (air-splint or canvas splint) it must be removed sufficiently so that everything below the splint can be saturated with the 0.5% CI solution. The patient, his wounds, and the decontaminable stretcher have now been completely deconned.

15. Final monitoring and movement to treatment area: The patient is monitored for contamination using chemical agent detection equipment. The contents of the M258A1 kit (pad 1 and pad 2 when used separately or together) and hypochlorite on the skin do not affect most detection devices. Once the casualty is confirmed clean of chemical agent he is transferred via a shuffle pit over the hot line. The shuffle pit is composed of two parts Super Tropical Bleach (STB) and 3 parts earth or sand. The shuffle pit should be deep enough to cover the bottom of the protective overboots. The buddy system wash of the TAP apron and gloves in 5.0% hypochlorite solution precedes the transfer of the patient to a new clean canvas litter if the decontaminable stretchers are in limited supply. A three-person patient lift is again used as the litter is switched. If the litter as well as the patient was checked, both patient and the same litter can be placed over the hot line.

7. **Decontamination procedure for ambulatory patient**

Decontamination of ambulatory patients follow the same principles as for litter patients. The major difference is the sequence of clothing removal, listed below, to lessen the chance of patient contaminating himself and others.

The first five steps are the same as in litter patient decontamination and are not described in detail.

1. Remove casualty's equipment.
2. Decontaminate mask and hood and remove hood.
3. Decontaminate skin around mask.
4. Remove Field Medical Card (triage tag) and put it into a plastic bag.
5. Remove gross contamination from the outergarment
   a. Remove and bag personal effects from overgarment.
6. Overgarment Jacket Removal

a. Instruct patient to:
   (1) Clench his fist.
   (2) Stand with arms held straight down.
   (3) Extend arms backward at about a 30 degree angle.
   (4) Place feet shoulder width apart.
b. Stand in front of patient.
   (1) Untie drawstring.
   (2) Unsnap jacket front flap.
   (3) Unzip jacket front.
c. Move to the rear of the patient.
   (1) Grasp jacket collar at sides of the neck.
   (2) Peel jacket off shoulders at a 30 degree angle down and away from the patient.
   (3) Smoothly pull the inside of sleeves over the patient's wrists and hands.
d. Cut to aid removal if necessary.

7. Removal of Butyl Rubber Gloves
   a. Patient's arms are still extended backward at a 30 degree angle.
      (1) Dip your gloved hands in 5% hypochlorite solution.
      (2) Use thumbs and forefingers of both hands.
         (a) Grasp the heel of patient's glove at top and bottom of forearm.
         (b) Peel gloves off with a smooth downward motion. This procedure can easily be done with one person or with one person on each side of the patient working simultaneously.
         (c) Place gloves in contaminated disposal bag.
   b. Tell the patient to reposition his arms, but not to touch his trousers.

8. Remove patient's overboots.
   a. Cut overboot laces with scissors dipped in 5% hypochlorite.
   b. Fold lacing eyelets flat on ground.
   c. Step on the toe and heel eyelet to hold eyelets on the ground.
   d. Instruct the patient to step out of the overboot onto clean area. If in good condition, the overboot can be decontaminated and reissued.

9. Remove overgarment trousers.
   a. Unfasten or cut all ties, buttons, or zippers.
   b. Grasp trousers at waist.
   c. Peel trousers down over the patient's boots.
   d. Cut trousers to aid removal if necessary.
      (1) Cut around all bandages and tourniquets.
      (2) Cut from inside pant leg ankle to groin.
      (3) Cut up both sides of the zipper to the waist.
      (4) Allow the narrow strip with zipper to drop between the legs.
      (5) Peel or allow trouser halves to drop to the ground.
   e. Tell patient to step out of trouser legs one at a time.
   f. Place trousers into contaminated disposal bag.

10. Remove glove inner liners. Patient should remove the liners since this will reduce the possibility of spreading contamination.

a. Tell patient to remove white glove liners.
    (1) Grasp heel of glove without touching exposed skin.
    (2) Peel liner downward and off.
    (3) Drop in contaminated disposal.
    (4) Remove the remaining liner in the same manner.
    (5) Place liners into contaminated disposal bag.
11. Final monitoring and decontamination
    a. Monitor/test with M8 Detection Paper or CAM.
    b. Check all areas of patient's clothing.
    c. Give particular attention to
        (1) Discolored areas
        (2) Damp spots
        (3) Tears in clothing
        (4) Neck
        (5) Wrist
        (6) around dressings
    d. Decontaminate all contamination on clothing or skin by cutting away areas of clothing or using 5% hypochlorite solution, the M291, or the M258A1 for clothing or 0.5% hypochlorite and the M291, or the M258A1 for skin.
12. The medic should remove bandages and tourniquets and decontaminate splints, using the procedures described in the decontamination of a litter patient, during overgarment removal.
13. The patient is decontaminated and ready to be moved inside the hot line. Instruct patient to shuffle his feet to dust his boots thoroughly as he walks through the shuffle pit.

In the clean treatment area the patient can now be re-triaged, treated, evacuated, etc. In a hot climate the patient will probably be significantly dehydrated and the rehydration process should start.

The clean area is the resupply point for the patient decontamination site. Water is needed for rehydration of persons working in the decon area. The resupply section should have an adequate stock of canteens with the chemical cap.

A location is needed in each decon area (75 meters from the working decon site) to allow workers, after they have deconned their TAP aprons, to remove their masks and rehydrate. There are generally not enough BDOs available to allow workers to remove them during the rest cycle and don new gear before going back to work. If these clean/shaded rest areas are not provided, the workers must remain fully dressed in protective ensembles even during rest periods, and water must be drunk through the mask via the drinking port. If all water consumption is by mask there must be a canteen refill area adjacent to the vapor/clean line in which empty canteens can be deconned and placed for refill and clean full canteens are present for rehydration.

8. Administering the Mark I autoinjector
1. Position yourself near the patient's left thigh (this will make it easier to reach into his mask carrier).

NOTE: If the patient has already received three doses of antidote, proceed to step 7.

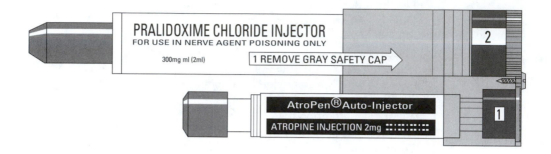

Figure B-12 Mark I Autoinjector.

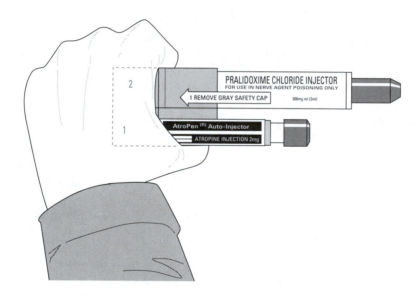

Figure B-13 Holding the set of injectors by the plastic clip.

2. Remove one set of antidote autoinjectors (Figure B-12) from the inside pocket of the patient's mask carrier.

NOTE: Do not use your autoinjector on a casualty. If you do, you may not have any antidote for self-aid.

3. Prepare to inject.
    a. Hold the set of injectors by the plastic clip (Figure B-13) with the big injector on top and in front of your body at eye level.
    b. Grasp the atropine autoinjector (the smaller of the two injectors) with your thumb and first two fingers of your other hand (Figure B-14).

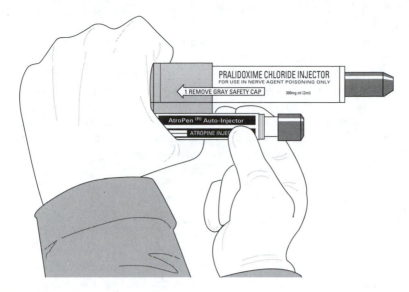

Figure B-14 Grasping the injectors.

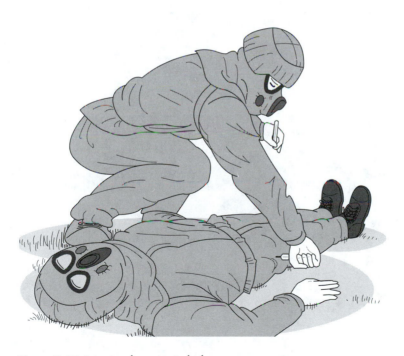

Figure B-15 Injecting the patient's thigh.

CAUTION Do not cover/hold the needle end with your hands or fingers - you may accidently inject yourself.

    c.   Pull the injector out of the clip with a smooth motion.

    d.   Form a fist around the injector.

4. Inject the atropine.

    a.   Place the green (needle) end of the injector against the patient's outer thigh muscle (Figure B-15).

    b.   Apply firm even pressure to the injector until it functions by pushing the needle into the patient's muscle, making sure you do not hit any objects in his pocket.

CAUTION Do not use a jabbing motion to inject the patient.

    c.   Hold the injector in place for at least **ten seconds** by counting one thousand one, one thousand two, and so forth.

    d.   Remove the injector.

CAUTION Watch out for the needle. Do not accidently inject yourself.

NOTE If the individual is very thin, you can inject him in the buttocks. Be careful to inject him only in the upper outer quadrant of the buttock (either side) because there is a nerve that crosses the buttocks and hitting this nerve can cause paralysis (Figure B-16).

    e.   Place the used injector carefully between the last two fingers of the hand that is holding the clip (Figure B-17).

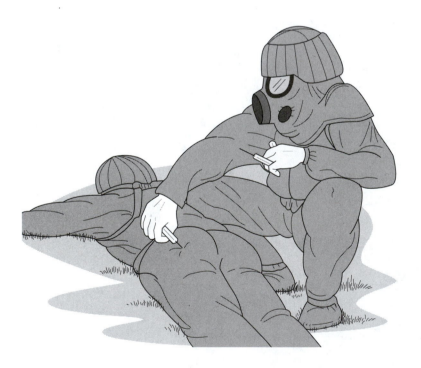

Figure B-16 Buttocks injection site. Be sure to inject in the upper outer quadrant of the buttock.

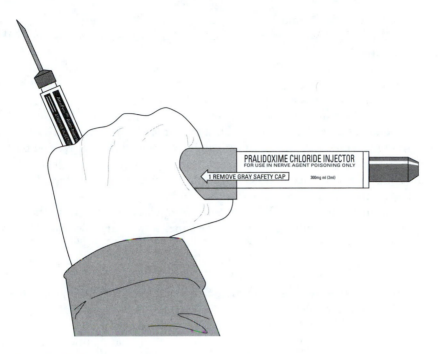

Figure B-17 Placing the used injector between the last two fingers.

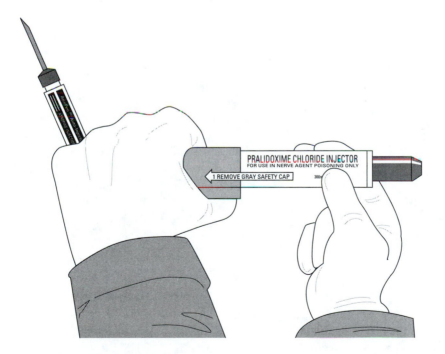

Figure B-18 Pulling out the 2 PAM Cl injector.

5. Inject the 2 PAM Chloride.
   a. Pull the 2 PAM Cl injector (the larger of the two injectors) from the clip (Figure B-18).
   b. Inject the patient in the same manner as for atropine previously, holding the black (needle) end against the patient's upper outer thigh (or buttock).
   c. Drop the clip without dropping the used injectors.
6. Attach the used autoinjectors to the patient's clothing [Note: This procedure is the traditional military method of marking a casualty as having received a Mark I kit. In light of universal precautions against handling contaminated sharps and the obvious risk of tearing your PPE, this procedure can no longer be recommended. Instead, dispose of the used injectors safely and note the administration of Mark I kit on the patient's triage tag or field medical card.]
   a. Pushing the needles of the used injectors, one at a time, through the left pocket flap. This will tell other medical personnel how many injectors were administered to the patient.
   b. Bend the needle to form a hook. Be careful not to tear your protective gloves while bending the needle.
7. Repeat the above steps, as appropriate for the patient's condition, using the second and third sets of antidote injectors.
8. Administer diazepam anticonvulsant using an autoinjector if the patient is having seizures or is symptomatic enough to require 3 sets of Mark I antidote autoinjectors.

Appendix C

FIELD AMPUTATION

Introduction

Field amputation is the surgical removal of a limb in order to free an otherwise hopelessly trapped victim. In essence, field amputation is the sacrifice of a limb to save a life. Field amputation should be a very rare event. However, the specter of widespread building collapse from explosive weapons of mass destruction mandate that prehospital personnel be familiar with this technique. It is the intent of this section to outline the use of field amputation and describe the basics of the procedure. It is not intended as a step-by-step guide to the performance of the procedure. Only physicians experienced in emergency procedures should perform field amputations (Table C-1). Prehospital personnel, however, play important roles in facilitating and assisting with the procedure, and should have a basic knowledge of its performance.

Because field amputation requires the direction and participation of a physician, community response plans should include a field amputation protocol. This protocol should address the personnel, equipment, transportation, and communication needs of bringing a qualified field amputation team to the scene. Inclusion of this team on disaster drills will help ensure a timely and effective response when called.

Indications

Field amputation is indicated for entrapped patients who are rapidly deteriorating and for whom rapid extrication is not possible. This is essentially the sacrifice of the limb to save

---

TABLE C-1

**REQUIREMENTS FOR PHYSICIANS AND ASSISTING PERSONNEL
TO PERFORM FIELD AMPUTATION**

Knowledge of the procedure
Familiar with confined-space rescue
Experienced in prehospital care environment
Committed and available

TABLE C-2

INDICATIONS FOR FIELD AMPUTATION IN ENTRAPPED PATIENTS

Rapidly deteriorating patient
Imminent threat from hazardous environment
Cannot extricate patient
Unsalvageable limb (relative indication)

a life (Table C-2). Another indication is an imminent and serious treat to the entrapped patient from a hazardous environment. Flames, fumes, rising water, and life-threatening hypothermia are possible hazards. Coordination with rescue and hazardous materials teams is essential to quantify the hazardous environment risk. Another possible indication is the hopelessly entrapped patient. Although the patient may not be imminently threatened, the possibility of a successful extrication may be so remote as to preclude reasonable hope. This may occur in large disasters where the infrastructure necessary to support a heavy extrication (e.g. cranes, bulldozers) may be destroyed or unavailable. In this case the decision to amputate should be made in conjunction with the teams responsible for heavy extrication. A relative indication for field amputation is an unsalvageable limb. The assessment of limb viability is difficult and cannot always be made with certainty in the field. Table C-3 lists the considerations when determining limb salvage.

Procedure

Field amputation requires some specialized equipment (Table C-4). Anesthesia and analgesia is critical. Several choices are available and Table C-5 lists several possibilities. Ketamine is favored because it does not depress respirations and rarely causes hypotension. Potential risks of ketamine include increased intracranial pressure and laryngospasm. Emergent hallucinations can be minimized with concomitant administration of moderate doses of a benzodiazepine. Narcotic analgesia is also a consideration since the procedure will likely be very painful. Advanced airway equipment should be readily available in the event of oversedation or airway compromise.

TABLE C-3

CONSIDERATIONS IN DETERMINING LIMB SALVAGE IN THE FIELD

Possibility of vascular repair
Possibility of skeletal repair
Viability of soft tissues
Viability of nervous function

TABLE C-4

EQUIPMENT CONSIDERATIONS FOR FIELD AMPUTATION

Bone saw, hand
Scalpels and handles (#10,11,20)
Clamps, small and medium Kelly
Absorbable and nonabsorbable suture
Needle drivers and pick-ups
Tourniquet
Betadine, sur-clens or similar cleanser
Adequate lighting
Gloves and personal protective gear
Airway management equipment
Sterile drapes, towels and dressings

TABLE C-5

MEDICATION CONSIDERATIONS FOR FIELD AMPUTATION

Anesthesia/Analgesia
    Ketamine
    Benzodiazepines (lorazepam, diazepam, midazolam)
    Narcotics (morphine, fentanyl)
Prophylactic Antibiotics/Antitoxins
    Cefazolin or similar-spectrum cephalosporin
    Tetanus-diphtheria

The patient should be fluid resuscitated as outlined under the crush injury section of Chapter 3, Care of Explosive and Incendiary Injuries. Oxygen therapy should be provided. Monitor the patient's vital signs every five minutes. Continuous ECG and pulse oximetry monitoring is desirable. Before beginning the procedure, prophylactic antibiotics and tetanus-diphtheria toxoid are administered. The anesthesia and analgesia administered should be sufficient for conscious sedation but not general anesthesia. Prep and drape the operative site as well as possible.

Field amputation for entrapped victims is carried out at the lowest possible anatomic level. Elevate the limb (if possible) and apply the tourniquet just above the site. Using the scalpel, the skin and soft tissue are divided down to the bone in a guillotine fashion. Clamp and tie any significant bleeders. Avoid incising the periosteum. Use the bone saw to transect the bone. Axial traction on the limb and smooth strokes on the saw will allow for a clean cut. Pack the amputated end of the limb with a pressure dressing and release the tourniquet. Transport the patient immediately to a facility with orthopedic surgical capability as the amputation will likely require revision.

If time and anatomy permit, plan the amputation with skin flaps in mind to cover the stump. Additionally, techniques other than a guillotine amputation may be preferred in some circumstances, particularly when transecting through joints.

Summary

Field amputation is a rare but potentially life-saving procedure. Communities should have a plan in place to provide this service if necessary. Prehospital providers should be familiar with the field amputation resources available and be prepared to assist on this procedure.